Thyroid Disease

Recent Titles in the Biographies of Disease Series

Rabies
P. Dileep Kumar

Influenza
Roni K. Devlin

ADHD
Paul Graves Hammerness

Food Allergies
Alice C. Richer

Anorexia
Stacy Beller Stryer

Obesity
Kathleen Y. Wolin, Sc.D. and Jennifer M. Petrelli

Sports Injuries
Jennifer A. Baima

Polio
Daniel J. Wilson

Cancer
Susan Elaine Pories, Marsha A. Moses, and Margaret M. Lotz

Fibromyalgia
Kim D. Jones and Janice H. Hoffman

Alcoholism
Maria Gifford

Anxiety
Cheryl Winning Ghinassi

Thyroid Disease

Sareh Parangi and Roy Phitayakorn

Biographies of Disease
Julie K. Silver, M.D., Series Editor

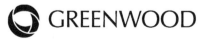 GREENWOOD

AN IMPRINT OF ABC-CLIO, LLC
Santa Barbara, California • Denver, Colorado • Oxford, England

Library of Congress Cataloging-in-Publication Data

Parangi, Sareh.
   Thyroid disease / Sareh Parangi and Roy Phitayakorn.
     p. ; cm. — (Biographies of disease)
   Includes bibliographical references and index.
   ISBN 978–0–313–37249–0 (hardcopy : alk. paper) — ISBN 978–0–313–37455–5
   (e-ISBN)
1. Thyroid gland—Diseases. I. Phitayakorn, Roy. II. Title. III. Series: Biographies of disease.
   [DNLM: 1. Thyroid Diseases. WK 200]
RC655.P34   2011
616.4′4—dc22   2010036284

ISBN: 978–0–313–37249–0
EISBN: 978–0–313–37455–5

15 14 13 12 11   1 2 3 4 5

This book is also available on the World Wide Web as an eBook.
Visit www.abc-clio.com for details.

Greenwood
An Imprint of ABC-CLIO, LLC

ABC-CLIO, LLC
130 Cremona Drive, P.O. Box 1911
Santa Barbara, California 93116-1911

This book is printed on acid-free paper ∞

Manufactured in the United States of America

Contents

Series Foreword

E very disease has a story to tell: about how it started long ago and began to disable or even take the lives of its innocent victims, about the way it hurts us, and about how we are trying to stop it. In this Biographies of Disease series, the authors tell the stories of the diseases that we have come to know and dread.

The stories of these diseases have all of the components that make for great literature. There is incredible drama played out in real-life scenes from the past, present, and future. You'll read about how men and women of science stumbled trying to save the lives of those they aimed to protect. Turn the pages and you'll also learn about the amazing success of those who fought for health and won, often saving thousands of lives in the process.

If you don't want to be a health professional or research scientist now, when you finish this book you may think differently. The men and women in this book are heroes who often risked their own lives to save or improve ours. This is the biography of a disease, but it is also the story of real people who made incredible sacrifices to stop it in its tracks.

Julie K. Silver, M.D.
Assistant Professor, Harvard Medical School
Department of Physical Medicine and Rehabilitation

Introduction

The human body is a real work of art and the more one learns about the details of its function, the more awed one becomes. The thyroid gland is a perfect example of the magnificence of the human body and physiology. The thyroid is a small hormone producing gland in the body that produces just one important hormone—*thyroid hormone*. It is remarkable that this tiny gland no bigger than the size of an adult's thumb can be so important for the proper function of the human body. The proper function of this small gland is important for the human body and mind to work correctly. People normally don't think of their thyroid, and those who know about it have either heard of it through their family members or from their doctors. Given the importance of the thyroid gland and the fact that over ten million Americans have thyroid diseases and over 37,000 had thyroid cancer last year, most people young or old will hear about the thyroid gland sooner or later in their lives. Some people first hear of this gland if their physician notes that their neck is thicker indicating an enlarged gland or there is a small lump found when the doctor feels their neck as part of their annual check-up. Others first hear of the thyroid gland when their friends refer to the thyroid as the gland in the neck that when not working properly, leads to obesity. And yet others first hear of the thyroid when a family member develops thyroid cancer. Even if you have never heard of the thyroid,

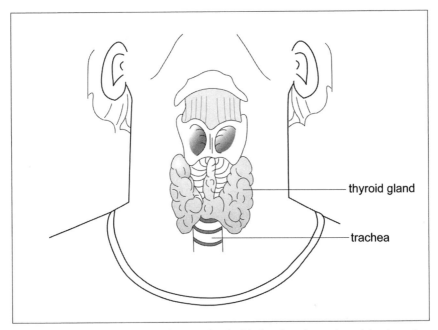

Figure I.1   A greatly simplified drawing that highlights the relationship of the thyroid to the rest of the neck. (Drawn by Sandy Windelspecht)

this book will take you on an informational journey about the role of this incredible gland. Keeping the thyroid healthy is important to the entire body and we will tell you the critical bits of information which will help you learn about this important gland and will guide you in keeping your own gland healthy.

The thyroid gland is a fairly small gland but it has a prominent place in the front part of a person's neck sitting just directly under the larynx or Adam's apple. This small gland is shaped like a butterfly and has three basic anatomic sections: The right lobe, the left lobe, and the middle connecting part called the isthmus (see Figure I.1). All three parts of the thyroid are functionally linked and work together to produce hormones.

Hormones are special chemical secreted from cells or organs that regulate the function of other tissues or organs. Thyroid hormone is a particularly important hormone and is really considered one of the key hormones that help all cells in the body run properly. Thyroid hormone controls how the *metabolism* of individual cells in the body works; each cell in the body maintains perfect efficiency in how it converts available nutrients into energy based on many factors but thyroid hormone appears to be one of the most important. Brain cells, muscle cells, heart cells, nerve cells. . . . in fact virtually every cell in the body relies on thyroid hormone to know how to properly function. So it is no surprise that when something happens to the fine-tuned function of the thyroid gland, all hell can break loose in the body. Each person's thyroid hormone level is regulated to a level that is comfortable and just right for them and keeps all the machinery in the body working well. If there is a problem with your home's thermostat or furnace, the house can become too hot or too cold. The same is true for the thyroid.

Too much thyroid hormone, hyperthyroidism, can lead an increased metabolic rate and increased heat production. This overactive thyroid can result in an increased metabolism, weight loss, heart palpitations, shaky hands, and constant sweating. This small gland can sure rev things up and make it seems like you are living in the fast lane all the time. Imagine if your home's thermostat was stuck in the on position, no matter how hot it got, it kept activating your furnace to turn on and produce more heat. Or imagine if your furnace was broken and no longer listened to the signals from your thermostat and just always stayed on no matter how hot your house got. As you can imagine, your house would become unbearably hot. This is exactly what happens when the signals to the thyroid, from a small gland in the brain, are way off or if the thyroid itself is stuck in an overproducing mode. . . . the thyroid just stays activated all the time, making too much thyroid hormone and the results can be dramatic and even deadly. U.S. President George H. W. Bush sure thought so when he was diagnosed with hyperthyroidism during the first Gulf War in 1991. When the thyroid gland of a sitting U.S. president acts up, it sure gets noticed!

The opposite can also happen where thyroid production drops off or stops completely, this condition is called *hypothyroidism*. Boy, things can sure slow down when that happens. Most people become hypothyroid because a critical mineral called iodine is missing or at very low levels in their everyday foods or their own immune system starts attacking their thyroid. People with hypothyroidism can slow down to a snail's pace. Too little circulating hormone causes their cells to become sluggish. The heart rate slows, the skin becomes dry and scaly, eyes can become puffy, energy levels are very low and the mind can become slow. When this happens to adults it can be magically reversed with the administration of thyroid hormone. Unfortunately in young infants the story is much worse. If a baby has a low functioning thyroid that is not diagnosed expertly and quickly, there can be permanent problems with bone and brain development. This can lead to significantly shorter stature and mental retardation. Read on and shortly you will see how the important link between one molecule (iodine), the gland that processes it (the thyroid) into an important molecule (thyroid hormone) and was eventually tied to *cretinism*—a severe form of mental and physical retardation that was affecting millions of children worldwide for millennia. Read on and you will find out about important worldwide efforts to use iodine supplementation to prevent and reverse mental retardation. Who would have thought a cheap and easy to produce mineral could prevent and cure some forms of mental retardation?

Deeper in the book you will leave the problems of the thyroid that are functional and will gain insight into what kinds of anatomic things can go wrong with the thyroid. Lumps, bumps, goiters, nodules, cysts, and cancers. ... you will learn about all these things. This book will cover it all, how to recognize them and how to treat them.

Most goiters start out as painless symmetric enlargements of the thyroid and when small, it is barely noticed by the person and no treatment is needed. Very large goiters can look cosmetically unappealing when they stick out in the neck and can be seen across the room. Some can get so large they can even block blood flow draining out of the head and neck causing the head and neck to get red and swell up. As goiters enlarge they can form *thyroid nodules* which are essentially lumps in the thyroid. These nodules can grow and squeeze the windpipe which sits under the thyroid, or in some rare cases, the thyroid cells in the nodules can become cancerous.

Thyroid cancers are generally rare compared to some other cancers such as lung or breast but the incidence is increasing. We will focus on discussing the differences and similarities between the different kinds of thyroid cancer (papillary, follicular, anaplastic, medullary, lymphoma, and rarer kinds). After reading the chapters on thyroid cancer and current research strategies you will see where the future of thyroid cancer research and therapies is going. You will be better armed to understand how thyroid cancer is different than other common cancers in humans and what is unique to the diagnosis and treatment of thyroid cancer. I think you will agree, doctors and researcher studying thyroid cancer have contributed immensely to the cancer field overall, even developing the first targeted therapy for cancer, radioactive iodine.

You will read about thyroid surgery and how it is used to treat both benign conditions of the thyroid when nothing else seems to be working and also how surgery is used to treat thyroid cancer. Hopefully you will find the sections on the history of thyroid surgery fascinating, who wouldn't? Can you imagine a surgical procedure that a mere 100 years ago results in at least 40 percent of the patients dying within a few days ... and now the mortality from thyroid surgery practically approaches zero? Read on and you will read about the surgical giants and medical heroes who managed this revolutionary change.

We hope you enjoy this book, but remember it is just a starting point. There is always more to know. Keep in mind that some people study the thyroid gland for a lifetime. The reference section in each chapter points you to important original work on the thyroid gland. Look up some of these sources online or in the library and your knowledge will be that much richer than your fellow students. Additional resources have been placed in the back of the book. Some of the listed organizations have incredible Web sites and informational packets, and for those who can't imagine life without Twitter or Facebook, there is even something for you since many of these sites are also on interactive social media.

1

Historical Perspectives on Thyroid Disease

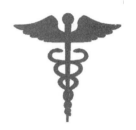

The history of medicine is not only fascinating but is also very important to study. It makes for fascinating reading and we urge every reader of this book to delve into the history of medicine as one of those uniquely exciting fields. The thyroid gland has played a prominent role in the history of medicine. Even quite early in many of the ancient texts on human diseases, forms of thyroid diseases are mentioned. It is fairly certain that a few aspects of thyroid disease were recognized as important in ancient times: *goiters, cretinism,* and the importance of *iodine* to the proper function of the thyroid. So we will talk about these two terms early on so there is a clearer understanding of their historic roles.

A thyroid goiter is basically an enlarged thyroid gland. When the thyroid enlarges, it can often be felt to be enlarged by the person themselves and can results in some pressure in the neck. If the thyroid enlarges even more, it has nowhere to go so it sticks out and becomes quite visible to the naked eye. It can even start pushing its way into the chest by crawling under the collar bone (*sub-sternal goiter*).

Cretinisim is a form of physical and mental retardation that can be caused by a less than normal amount of thyroid hormone. The term cretin was first used in 1754 in *Diderot's Encylopedie* and referred to a mentally handicapped man who was deaf and dumb and had a goiter hanging down to his waist. It turns out proper function of the thyroid is very important to development of the brain, muscles, bones, and all other aspects of a growing human child. Deficiency in thyroid hormone (from any cause) during critical phases of a child's development can lead to permanent mental and developmental delays. The medical and sociological implications of cretinism due to thyroid hormone deficiency is seen the world over. Indeed, just the term cretinism or cretin obviously has a negative social connotation due to the slow mental processes of the person afflicted with this condition. In this chapter, you will surely see the slow evolution of how lay people, healers, doctors, and researchers slowly put the pieces of the puzzle together to make the important link between one molecule (iodine), the gland that processes it (the thyroid) into an important molecule (thyroid hormone), and made the tremendously important connections to cretinism—a severe form of mental and physical retardation that was affecting millions of children worldwide for millennia.

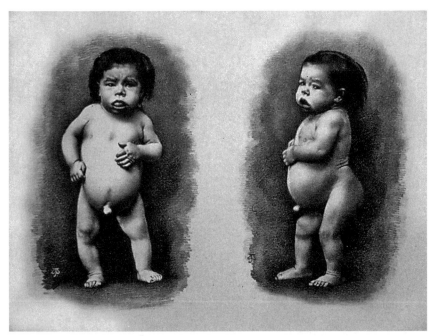

A photograph of a child in the late 1800s with cretinism due to severe hypothyroidism showing coarse features, short stature, and mental retardation. (National Library of Medicine)

IODINE DEFICIENCY AND GOITER: AN ANCIENT SCOURGE

Chinese physicians of the Tang dynasty (618–907 AD) were the first to give the iodine rich thyroid glands from animals such as sheep and pigs in dried and powdered forms or mixed into wine to treat people with goiters (Temple 1986). Between 1000 and 1100 AD, two Persian physicians, Avicenna and later Zayn al-Din-al-Jurani, first described the association of goiter and bulging of the eyes (*exopthalmus*) in the *Cannon of Medicine*, a medical textbook, this is the first description of a patient with goiter and Graves' disease (Nabipour, Burger et al. 2009). Paracelus (1493–1541) was the first to propose a relationship between minerals like lead in the drinking water and goiter formation. Iodine was later discovered in Paris by Bernard Courtois in 1811 from seaweed ash (Markel 1987). The Swiss physician Coindet successfully treated patients with goiter using tincture of iodine in 1821. By 1894, Baumann had discovered that iodine was present in the normal thyroid gland at markedly higher concentrations than in thyroid goiters (Baumann and Roos 1896). Perhaps the most important links between iodine and thyroid came from Dr. David Marine and his collaborators in Ohio (see Figure 1.1). With a little detective work, he deducted through his experiments on the thyroids of trout between 1910 and 1917 that giving school age girls iodine would prevent thyroid enlargement: 2,200 girls were treated with iodine for two years and only 5 developed goiters; 2,300 were not treated and almost 500 developed thyroid enlargement (Marine and Kimball 1917). These impressive findings led to a flurry of efforts in the United States and Europe and public health workers. The Swiss recommended using iodized salt in 1922 and in Rochester, N.Y., sodium iodide was put into the town drinking water a year later.

IODINE DEFICIENCY: WORLD WAR I AND THE DISCOVERY OF THE U.S. GOITER BELT

The iodine deficiency problem in the United States really came to wide public attention when World War I started. During the 1918 draft registration it became obvious that in the Michigan region, 30 percent of all male recruits were disqualified because of a large goiter, decreased mentation, and major physiologic issues. Just in Northern Michigan alone, over 20,000 young men were disqualified for service. Well, this sure got everyone's attention and soon a wide area of Michigan was listed as being in the "goiter belt" with a striking deficiency in iodine in both water and soil. Soon the Michigan State Medical Society became involved and eventually it was decided that the best way to make sure everyone in Michigan had access to enough iodine to prevent goiter, was to add small quantities of sodium iodide to table salt.

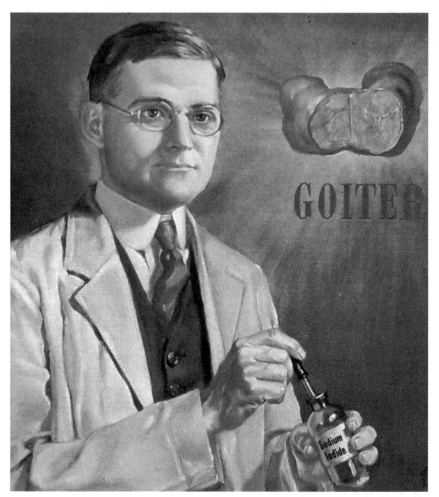

Dr. David Marine (1888–1976) was an American pathologist who discovered that iodine supplementation prevented goiters. His research ultimately led to the iodinization of table salt. (National Library of Medicine)

IODIZATION OF SALT: WHEN IT RAINS IT POURS

Who would think to add iodine to salt and why was salt chosen? Salt was chosen as the quickest most efficient means to combat the huge problem of goiter because of some pretty simple but nifty reasoning. Salt is produced in large quantities by just a few companies, everyone consumes it, adding iodine does not change its taste, color, or odor and it is cheap to do. It costs less than half a cent to iodize one kilogram (approximately a half pound) of salt! Iodized salt was first produced by Diamond Crystal Salt in 1924 and four months later The Morton Salt Company started selling iodized salt all over the United States. By 1932, over 90 percent of the salt sold in Michigan was iodized. Wow, what a quick transition.

Iodized salt became quickly popular all over the United States with scientific studies showing its efficacy in preventing endemic goiter. There were some naysayers initially though, and some pretty prominent ones at that too. For example, Dr. Emil Kocher who had won the Nobel Prize in 1909 for his work on the physiology and surgery of the thyroid gland emphatically denied therapy with iodine and thought it would lead to hyperthyroidism. In fact, it was thought that Dr. Kocher would dismiss any surgical assistant who even dared to use iodine to wash the skin of his patients prior to thyroid surgery (McClure 1934).

IODINE DEFICIENCY AND CRETINISM: MOST COMMON CAUSE OF PREVENTABLE MENTAL RETARDATION

Iodine deficiency is now considered the most common cause of preventable brain damage in the world today (World Health Organization 2002), but this association has not always been clear. The problem has arisen because for thousands of years, people have lived in an environment where the soil has been leached of the mineral iodine through erosion, as well as flooding. This poor soil then leads to low levels of iodine in all the grains and cereals that grow on that soil, as well as in the animals that feed on it. Humans cannot form the mineral, and yet it is essential for human brain development because iodine is the building block of thyroid hormone.

The relation between iodine deficiency and brain damage was originally raised by observing the association that some people with severe mental retardation had large goiters, probably in the medieval times, though records of goiters date back to at least 3000 BC. The term cretin was first used in *Diderot's Encylopedie* in 1754 and referred to an imbecile who was deaf and dumb and had a goiter hanging down to his waist. This was a condition seen commonly at that time in the mountainous regions of Europe, such as Switzerland, France, and northern Italy. In 1848, the King of Sardinia helped fund and publish an epidemiologic survey on cretinism in the European Alps. Not much attention was paid to the cause of cretinism until the 1930–1960s when descriptions of it began appearing again in the medical literature and a clear syndrome was described. Endemic cretinism can be severe with brain damage, mutism and severe muscle spasms. Milder forms of cretinism occurred when there was severe iodine deficiency in late pregnancy resulting in short stature and brain damage. The link between iodine and cretinism was confirmed in the 1960 when countries such as Papua New Guinea started injecting poppy seed oil containing iodine supplements to correct iodine deficiency. These injections supplied the person with four years of adequate iodine intake. When women of childbearing age where injected in large groups, the rates of stillbirths and cretinism fell dramatically. It then became widely accepted worldwide that the iodine deficiency was the main reason that these children had developed cretinism. This was an amazing discovery and the World Health Organization (WHO) labeled iodine deficiency as the single most important cause for mental retardation worldwide. The WHO then dedicated itself to eliminating iodine deficiency through an intense program to iodize salt. This heroic effort is ongoing and once complete will be on the scale of other worldwide public health triumphs such as the eradication of small pox and polio. The amount of iodine needed by each person for their entire lifetime is less than one teaspoon, supplying all humans with this would cost less than five cents per person per year. Obviously this is much less than the cost to society that incurs in taking care of one person with severe mental retardation due to iodine deficiency (see Figure 1.1).

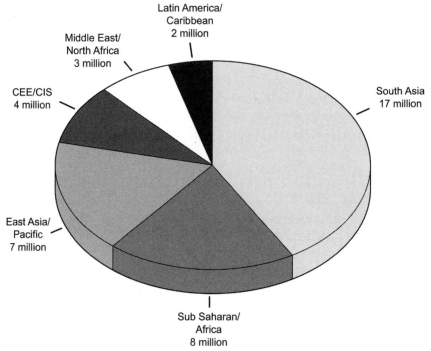

Figure 1.1   Iodine deficiency remains a major source of learning disabilities worldwide. (World Health Organization)

Keep in mind that there is a graded effect of iodine deficiency on the brain. Ten percent have severe iodine deficiency and suffer from the symptoms of cretinism described above. Thirty percent have less severe brain damage but have lowered intelligence upon testing. Between 60 and 70 percent may have loss of mental and physical energy due to low thyroid hormone levels caused by mild to moderate deficiency in iodine, this condition is reversible and can be quite dramatic by supplementation of the diet with iodine as there is no permanent brain damage in these individuals.

IODINE: HOW MUCH IS ENOUGH?

Iodine is found in many different food sources including iodized salt, iodinized bread, fortified dairy products, shellfish, white deep-water fish, brown seaweed kelp, garlic, lima beans, sesame seeds, spinach, Swiss chard, summer squash, and turnip greens. Iodine can also be found in radio contrast materials, topical antiseptics such as povidone-iodine, and medications such as amiodarone. The recommended daily amount of iodine is listed in the Table 1.1.

Some people have just the right amount of iodine in the foods they eat on a daily basis. However, some people eat diets rich in certain foods which block the body's ability to absorb iodine, such as cassava root or soybeans. Eating lots of these "goiterogens" in the food leads to thyroid goiter formation. Taking in food or medications with too much iodine can cause hyperthyroidism, especially

Table 1.1
Recommended Daily Amount of Iodine

Pediatric

For infants ages 0–6 months: The recommended daily amount of iodine is 40 micrograms (mcg).

For infants ages 6 months to 1 year: The recommended daily amount of iodine is 50 mcg.

For children ages 1–10 years: The recommended daily amount of iodine is 70–120 mcg.

For children ages 10–18 years: The recommended daily amount of iodine is 120–150 mcg.

Adult

For males and females 18 years and up: The recommended daily amount of iodine is 120–150 mcg.

For pregnant females: The recommended daily amount of iodine is 175 mcg.

For lactating and breast-feeding females: The recommended daily amount of iodine is 200 mcg.

Source: Food and Nutrition Board of the U.S. National Academy of Sciences.

if a person's thyroid was already under constant Thyroid-Stimulating Hormone (TSH) stimulation. For example, Dr. Carl von Basedow noted that giving someone iodine when they previously had baseline iodine deficiency can trigger severe episodes of hyperthyroidism. This phenomenon is called the Jod-Basedow phenomenon (*Jod* means iodine in German). Laboratory evaluation in a person who has hyperthyroidism from excessive iodine, typically demonstrates increased levels of plasma thyroglobulin, iodine, and thyroid hormone levels. Discontinuation of the offending agent is the treatment of choice and symptomatic therapy with a beta-blocker medication may be helpful.

PUBLIC HEALTH MEASURES TO PREVENT GOITER AND MENTAL RETARDATION: NOW THAT'S PROGRESS!

Iodide or Iodate, which are more stable forms of iodine have now been used for more than 80 years as an additive to table salt as a public health measure. Extensive national and international programs have been put in place; this has not been cheap or easy. Commitment from industry, governments, and nongovernmental organizations all over the world has led to a safe and reliable way to deliver much needed iodine all over the world, even to some pretty remote places. The World Health Organization and UNICEF are the biggest supporters of this global battle. At the end of the twentieth century, 68 percent of households in the world had access to iodized salt, with some areas at over 90 percent such as the Americas. This herculean effort has ensured that 80 million newborns have better mental and physical health and increased the overall IQ of the world by over one billion points! However, there are still at least 41 million newborns who are not protected' and global partnerships are hard at work today to eliminate iodine deficiency once and for all as the cause of goiter and mental retardation worldwide (Hetzel 2004).

REFERENCES

Baumann, E., and E. Roos (1896). "Ueber das normale Vorkommen des Jods im thierkorper." *Ztschr f Physiol Chem* **21**: 481.

Hetzel, B. S., Ed. (2004). *Towards the Global Elimination of Brain Damage Due to Iodine Deficiency*. Delhi, Oxford University Press.

Marine, D., and O. P. Kimball (1917). "The prevention of simple goiter in man." *J. Lab Clin Medicine* **3**: 40–43.

Markel, H. (1987). " 'When it rains it pours': endemic goiter, iodized salt, and David Murray Cowie, MD." *Am J Public Health* **77**(2): 219–29.

McClure, R. D. (1934). "Thyroid surgery in southern Michigan as affected by the generalized use of iodized salt." *J. Michigan State Medical Society* **33**: 58–62.

Nabipour, I., A. Burger, et al. (2009). "Avicenna, the first to describe thyroid-related orbitopathy." *Thyroid* **19**(1): 7–8.

Temple, R. (1986). *The Genius of China: 3000 Years of Science, Discovery, and Invention.* New York, Simon and Shuster, Inc.

World Health Organization. (2002). "Mortality and burden of disease estimates for WHO member States" from http://www.who.int/entity/healthinfo/statistics/bodgbddeath dalyestimates.xls.

2

The Thyroid Gland

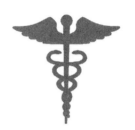

THYROID ANATOMY: WHERE IS THE THYROID ANYWAY?

The thyroid sits in the anterior part of the neck and is one of the few endocrine organs that can be felt by people themselves, as well as physicians on physical examination. Enlargement of the thyroid, lumps, or tumors of the thyroid gland will often be noticed by the patient or the examining physician. Thyroid cells in the fetus develop at the base of the tongue, and as the fetus matures, the thyroid slowly divides into two lobes, acquiring the shape of a shield and moving downward to the neck where it is found just below the Adam's apple in most people. The neck is a narrow channel through which many important structures pass to the rest of the body such as the food pipe (esophagus), the windpipe (trachea), the arteries supplying blood to the brain (carotid arteries), and veins bringing blood back from the brain (jugular veins) as well as the spinal cord, the voice box, and many important nerves. The thyroid is intricately placed among these structures right on top of the windpipe and next to the food pipe. If the thyroid enlarges, it can squeeze these important structures and cause problems with breathing or swallowing. If the thyroid enlarges even more, it has nowhere to go so it sticks out and becomes visible as a *goiter* or can even start pushing its way into the chest by slowly growing under the collar bone (*sub-sternal goiter*).

Since the thyroid descends from its original location along the base of the tongue to the neck, there are some interesting anatomic variations or congenital abnormalities that can be seen in some people. Rarely, thyroid tissue can remain in its original position at the base of the tongue "lingual thyroid," where it can still grow and function normally, but can sometimes be mistaken for an overgrown tonsil or tumor in a child and be removed accidentally. Sometimes during descent into the neck other problems can occur when pieces of developing thyroid tissue can be left behind called *ectopic thyroid tissue*, or they can form small or large cysts in the neck that may get swollen or infected and need to be removed in early childhood—*thyroglossal ducts cysts*.

In most people, the thyroid correctly descends to its location in the front of the neck and sits directly underneath the superficial muscles of the neck. The thyroid has a very rich blood supply and has one of the highest amounts of blood flow in the body for its size, therefore surgery on the thyroid has to be done very meticulously to avoid drastic bleeding complications. This rich blood supply comes directly from the aorta, the largest blood vessel in the body, and it is very important to the function of the thyroid. The two main arteries that feed the thyroid are the *superior and inferior thyroid artery* (see Figure 2.1).

Two other structures are intimately associated with the thyroid gland. The nerves to the voice box, called the *Recurrent Laryngeal Nerves* (*RLN*), run behind the thyroid in a small groove on the way to the voice box. These nerves arise directly from one of the *cranial nerves* (*the Vagus* or the tenth cranial nerve). Pressure from an enlarged thyroid or tumor of the thyroid can affect these nerves by compressing them causing the voice to become hoarse. Most recurrent laryngeal nerves travel to the voice box in the same consistent pathways, but there can be some 50 different anatomic variations in the travel path of the nerve. Again, during thyroid surgery of any kind it is extremely important that the surgeon be extremely familiar with all these variations so as not to damage or stretch these nerves, since any damage to the nerve can significantly change the quality of the voice. The parathyroid glands are tiny lentil-sized glands that help regulate the body's calcium level. The four glands share a blood supply with the thyroid and sit behind the thyroid (see Figure 2.2).

THYROID PHYSIOLOGY: WHAT DOES THE THYROID DO?

The thyroid only has one function in life—to produce thyroid hormone at just the right amounts for each person. This seemingly simple task is actually quite complex and has been the topic of intense research for over 50 years. For the purposes of understanding the intricacy of the different organs involved in proper function of the thyroid, an analogy to a common household item

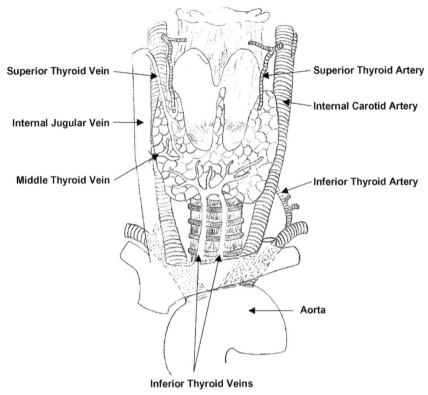

Figure 2.1   The thyroid gland is rich in blood supply. There are two feeding arteries and three draining veins. (Drawn by Dr. Jamie Mitchell, MD)

sometimes helps. Think of the thyroid as functioning like the furnace in a house. The thyroid produces thyroid hormone for release and use, just like a furnace produces heat and distributes it throughout the house. This furnace analogy will be helpful in understanding how the thyroid gland works and manages to put out just the right amount of thyroid hormone (see Table 2.1).

Although your thyroid does make thyroid hormone, how much it makes and how much it releases is under the regulation of a two small glands at the base of the brain called the *pituitary and hypothalamus*. The pituitary gland acts similar to the thermostat in your house. Let's say your house temperature is set at a comfortable 70 degrees in the winter. If the house environment is too cold and reaches 67 degrees, your thermostat senses that your house is too cold, it sends an electric signal to your house's furnace to start up and produce heat. Once the house reaches 70 degrees and is nice and cozy again, the thermostat no longer sends the activate signal to the furnace and the furnace shuts back down. The pituitary gland in the brain makes

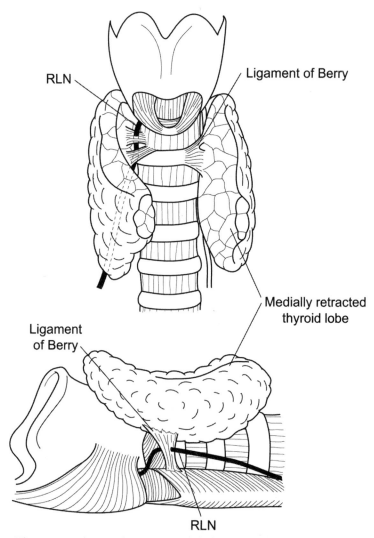

Figure 2.2   The recurrent laryngeal nerve passes behind the thyroid and is at risk during thyroid surgery. Injury to this nerve on one side can result in a hoarse whispery voice in some patients. (Drawn by Jeff Dixon after Randolph, 2003)

measurements of your thyroid hormone level on a daily basis acting similarly to your house's thermostat. When the pituitary senses that your thyroid hormone levels are too low for optimal functioning (the house is too cold), it sends a special hormonal signal called *Thyroid Stimulating Hormone* (TSH) into the bloodstream. This special signal arrives at the thyroid, "stimulates" the thyroid to start capturing more iodine,

Table 2.1
Furnace to Thyroid Comparison

House	Action in House	Human Body	Action in Body
Owner of the house	Sets temperature of thermostat	Hypothalamus	Master gland that sets body's thyroid hormone level
Thermostat	Detects that house is too cold and sends electric signal to turn on furnace	Pituitary gland	Sensor in the body that detects low thyroid hormone levels and secretes Thyroid Stimulating Hormone to turn on thyroid
Kick-start signal from thermostat	Electric signal arrives at furnace and kick-starts heat production	Thyroid Stimulating Hormone (TSH)	Hormone that travels in blood and acts to increases production of thyroid hormone from the thyroid
Furnace	Produces heat to increase temperature in house and maintain right temperature in the house	Thyroid Gland	Produces thyroid hormone to increase thyroid hormone levels and maintain right balance in the body

producing more thyroid hormone, and at the same time to release any stored thyroid hormone. As a result of this stimulation, the thyroid gland doubles up its thyroid hormone production and the level of thyroid hormone in the blood rises. Once a normal thyroid hormone level is achieved, the pituitary stops production of TSH and *homeostasis* is achieved, everything is just right again. The pinpoint precision of this "Negative Feedback Control System" is common in the body and is used in control of many other hormones as well. In fact the pituitary gland itself is under the control of the *Hypothalamus*, another important gland in the brain through a similar mechanism called the *Hypothalamic-Pituitary Axis*. The hypothalamus is a master controller of many of the hormone producing organs of the body, for the purposes of this analogy, it acts like the homeowner, setting the temperature of the house at the level it senses is right for each individual (see Figure 2.3).

IMPORTANCE OF HAVING A BALANCED THYROID HORMONE: NOT TOO HOT, NOT TOO COLD, JUST RIGHT ALL THE TIME ... WHEW, THAT IS HARD WORK

The thyroid helps regulate most aspects of the human body's physiology, through the regulation of just one hormone. It should not come as a shocker then that the thyroid has to run "just right" for everything to work smoothly in the body. Having

What History Can Teach Us:
Thyroid Surgery: Can It Ruin Your Singing?
The Case of Amelita Galli-Curci

Amelita Galli-Curci was an Italian opera singer who after her operatic debut in 1906, toured extensively around the world to great acclaim. Still relatively unknown in the United States in 1916, she created a sensation in the Chicago Opera's production of Verdi's *Rigoletto*, beginning her reign as an operatic star in New York and Chicago for more than a decade.

By the late 1920s, her voice was in decline and critics began commenting on flat notes and her strained singing, ultimately leading to her retirement in 1930. She met an American surgeon specializing in thyroid surgery in 1935, while on tour in India, she was noted to have a large goiter pushing on her trachea and was thought to be perhaps the reason for the more obvious vocal difficulty she had been having. When Galli-Curci returned to the United States, Dr. Arnold Kegel arranged to perform a thyroidectomy on August 11, 1935. The surgical procedure was performed under local anesthesia, and at several points during the surgery the surgeon asked the patient to sings so as to ensure that the laryngeal nerves were not traumatized. At the end, she sang part of a duet from *The Barber of Seville*. Her first vocal exercises were performed in the ward, and her voice was initially harsh.

When one of the nurses commented, "Wonderful, Madame," she replied acerbically, "Wonderful? It sounds like a buzz saw hitting a rusty nail!" Initially, she was a happy customer, claiming that removal of her "little potato in the throat" had helped her breathing and singing, and she tried to make a comeback after not singing opera for six years. At first the Chicago City Opera was excited about getting their star back, and cast her in an important starring role as Mimi in La Bohème. The performance in 1936 was a disaster and the critics harshly reviewed her, calling her voice "pathetic."

She eventually went on to blame the thyroid surgery and the surgeon for ending her operatic career in an important interview. Rather, it is likely that the improved airflow that followed the removal of the goiter imparted a sense of freedom that allowed her for a time to avoid confronting the fact that her voice had been declining steadily for several years. Given the evidence that her voice had been declining for years, it is likely that Dr. Kegel's thyroidectomy did not precipitate the end of Galli-Curci's career as a soprano, but this historical vignette is an important lessons for thyroid surgeons to take extra care around the larger recurrent laryngeal nerve and the smaller nerves such as the superficial laryngeal nerve which can affect voice quality (Crookes and Recabaren 2001).

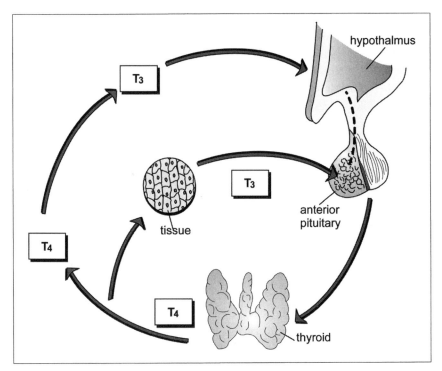

Figure 2.3   Regulation of thyroid hormone release from the thyroid is under the influence of a classic feedback loop involving the hypothalamus and pituitary glands in the brain. TRH from the hypothalamus triggers the secretion of TSH from the pituitary. TSH then stimulates the thyroid to increase production and release of thyroid hormone. Circulating levels of T4 and T3 influence the hypothalamus and pituitary to regulate thyroid hormone production. (Drawn by Sandy Windelspecht)

a balanced level of thyroid hormone is very important. We have to step back and look at how the thyroid keeps balanced, and then in later chapters, we will look at some problems that commonly develop if the amount of thyroid hormone in the body is not just right.

The thyroid cells sit in clusters called *follicles* in the organ. These follicles each are made of individual thyroid follicular cells which work together to produce thyroid hormone. The follicular cells are arranged like stones around a campfire. Inside each of the follicular cells, the extracted iodine is processed by a special enzyme called *thyroid peroxidase*, and is coupled with a special protein produced only inside thyroid cells called *thyroglobulin*. The iodine atoms are rapidly oxidized and covalently bound (*organified*) to specific tyrosine residues of thyroglobulin. The thyroglobulin and the iodine atoms are put together inside each cell to produce thyroid hormone. Some of the thyroid hormone is immediately secreted, but much of the hormone is stored in small pools called *colloid* in a central storage compartments (where the campfire would be) on the inside of each follicle until the body calls for more thyroid hormone. When the body needs thyroid hormone, the pituitary secretes the chemical signal TSH to rev up the thyroid and stored thyroid hormone is released and certain bloodstream proteins chaperone the thyroid hormone in the bloodstream and helps it get to all the critically important places in the body that need it. Thyroid hormone, like heat, is then delivered to the entire body (see Figure 2.5).

Each person's thyroid hormone level is regulated to a level that is comfortable and just right for them and keeps all the machinery in the body working well. If there is a problem with your home's thermostat or furnace, the house can become too hot or too cold. The same is true for the thyroid.

Having too much thyroid hormone can wreak havoc on the body, this condition is called *hyperthyroidism*. Imagine if your home's thermostat was stuck in the on position, no matter how hot it got, it kept activating your furnace to turn on and produce more thyroid hormone. Or imagine if your furnace was broken and no longer listened to the signals from your thermostat and just always stayed on no matter how hot your house got. As you can imagine, your house would become unbearably hot. If the anterior pituitary, the gland in the brain that acts as a thermostat, sends too much signal to your thyroid, causing it to always be in overdrive, the furnace makes too much heat. This means that your thyroid hormone concentration goes up, and the resulting "hyperthyroidism" causes and increased metabolic rate and increased heat production. You, like your house, will become overheated, very hot, and you will sweat a lot because of too much heat. This is exactly what happens when there is hyperthyroidism or overproduction of thyroid hormone. We will go over the various causes of hyperthyroidism in detail in the next chapter.

The opposite problem is called *hypothyroidism*. In this condition, the thyroid shuts off production of thyroid hormone either because it is malfunctioning or it receiving no stimulatory signals from the pituitary. You can imagine that if the furnace breaks down and there is no heat produced, the house will slowly get cold. This is exactly what happens in hypothyroidism; there is not enough thyroid hormone produced and the body starts slowing down at the cellular level. Too little thyroid hormone slows down the metabolism of all cells, but can have certain especially devastating effects. If thyroid hormone production is completely shut off during fetal development, and in the immediate newborn period, the baby will not grow normally. This condition known as *cretinism* results in severely diminished mental capacity and intelligence as well as significantly stunted physical development. We will next look at how the thyroid gland produces thyroid hormone and gets it to the rest of the body in just the right amounts.

One More Thing to Know: Now That's Interesting
Thyroid Physiology: Lessons from the Animal World
What Do Frogs Have to Do with Baby Bottles?

Do you remember your fascination when you first found out that frogs came from tadpoles? Surely you wondered how the tadpole knows when to change form into a mature frog? In the 1970s, researchers discovered that this metamorphosis was one more example of the powerful action of thyroid hormone. Thyroid hormone was the signal that made tadpoles transform into frogs and without this important physiologic signal for metamorphosis, tadpoles remained tadpoles (Cohen 1970). This was fascinating stuff and quite exciting that one single hormone could trigger such a massive transformation with changes in brain structure, bony structures, muscle, and caused important things like the tail of the tadpole to disappear. It was really quite remarkable. Over the next three decades, lots of details emerged about the importance of thyroid hormone on the brain development of human fetuses and infants as well. Soon people started asking questions about the effects of certain commonly used plastics such as Bisphenol A (BPA) which is often added to many plastics to make them more durable and help prevent them from breaking. BPA is found in many polycarbonate items such as water bottles, baby bottles, compact discs, and sports equipment. Since humans use these plastic products everyday, some amount of BPA is found in over 90 percent of humans, with higher levels in infants and children. In 2009 researchers working at the National Institute of Health (Heimeier, Das et al. 2009) discovered that exposing tadpoles to high levels of BPA can alter thyroid hormone levels and prevent proper development. This information from the tadpole world was then used to conclude that since proper thyroid hormone levels are very important for optimal development of the infant brain, it is best not to feed infants with baby bottles containing BPA. High BPA levels in the milk may lower thyroid hormone levels in the babies and results in delayed brain development. Thyroid hormone is important for frogs and humans. Until more definitive data is obtained, it's probably best to avoid toxins which might significantly change the thyroid hormone balance.

THYROID HORMONE PRODUCTION: LET'S GET SOME DETAILS HERE

Thyroid hormone production starts with extraction of a particular mineral called iodine from dietary sources. This is no simple task, because iodine is a trace mineral and found in fairly low quantities in the soil, water, and certain food items. When foods rich and iodine such as seafood, iodized salt, milk, and bread are eaten, the iodine is extracted from the food and travels in the blood-stream to the thyroid. As the blood flows through the thyroid, the thyroid cells themselves efficiently extract the iodine out of the bloodstream and into the cells themselves. Specialized receptors on the surface of thyroid cells called the *Sodium-Iodine Symporter* (NIS) work around the clock to pull iodine into the cell. The thyroid follicle acts as an independent mini factory for thyroid hormone and generally each cell in the follicle adds the extracted iodine to certain amino acids (building blocks of proteins) molecules and ultimately two important thy-roid hormones, *L-thyroxine* (T4) and *L-triiodothyronine* (T3), are produced. Three iodine atoms are used to make T3 and four iodine atoms are used to make T4. T3 is considered the biologically active hormone. Most actions of thyroid hormone happen when T3 binds to its nuclear receptors on many different cell types in the human body (see Figures 2.4 and 2.5).

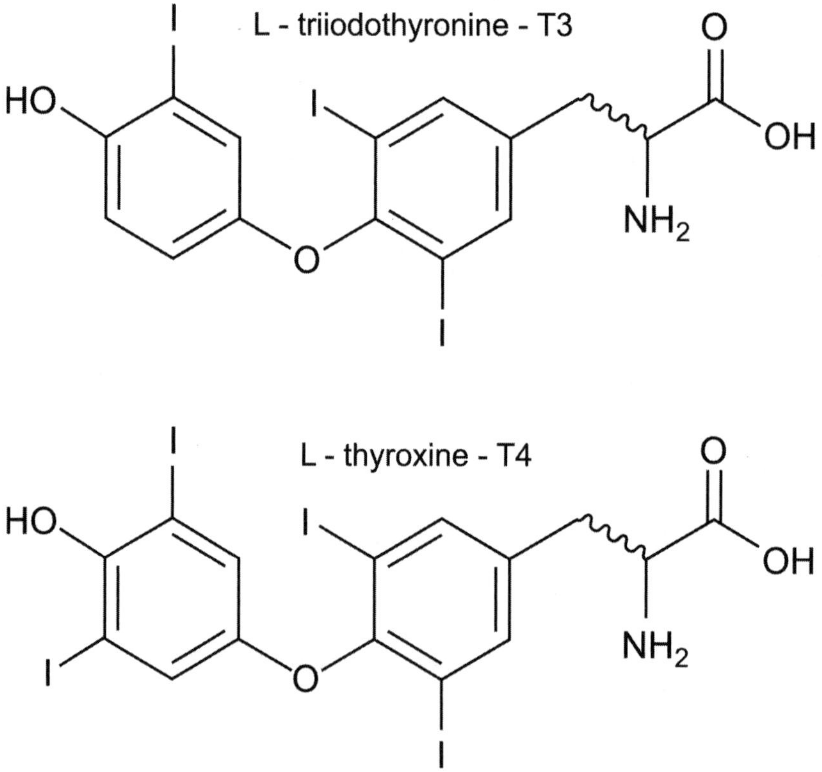

Figure 2.4   Thyroid hormones—T3 and T4. (Drawn by Jeff Dixon)

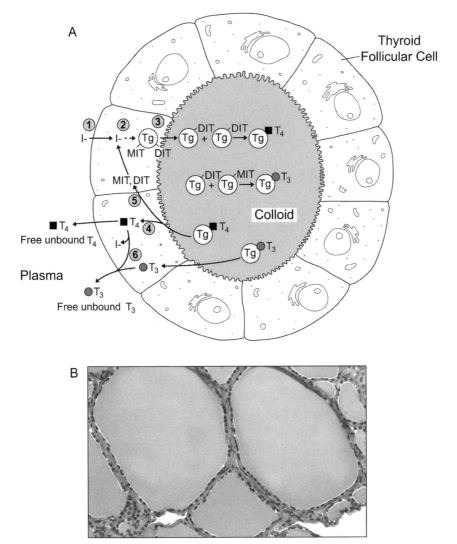

Figure 2.5 Production and storage of thyroid hormone in the thyroid gland. Panel A—the thyroid follicular cells form large follicles which help produce and store thyroid hormones (T4 and T3) in the thyroid gland. Panel B—reveals large thyroid follicular cells formed into macrofollicles. Thyroid hormone and colloid, seen as intense pink material stored at the center of each follicle, is released by the thyroid as needed. (Redrawn by Jeff Dixon after McPherson & Pincus: *Henry's Clinical Diagnosis and Management by Laboratory Methods*, 2006/Photo courtesy Dr. Sareh Parangi, MD)

The thyroid gland mostly produces T4 (around 90 mcg per day). Inside the thyroid there is only a tiny bit of T3 (6 mcg produced per day). Most of the secreted thyroid hormones gets safely chaperoned around the body by tightly binding to certain proteins such as *thyroid binding thyroglobulin* (TBG), *thyroid binding prealbumin,* or *albumin.* Once the T4 is secreted into the bloodstream, special proteins called *deiodinase enzymes* remove one of the four iodine atoms of T4 thus creating an abundance of T3 hormone in the peripheral organs such as the kidney, liver, and brain. Three enzymes catalyzing these deiodinations have been identified, called type 1 (D1), type 2 (D2), and type 3 (D3) *iodothyronine deiodinases.* These enzymes themselves use another rare mineral called *selenium* to enzymatically convert T4 to T3, the active form of thyroid hormone. D1 is expressed mainly in the liver, the kidneys, and the thyroid. D1 produced in the liver appears to be the principal enzyme converting most of the body's T4 to T3.D2 works mainly in fat and the central nervous system, and it is thought to mostly be important in micromanagement of the thyroid hormone level at local tissue levels. D3 is important in degradation of thyroid hormone and inactivates T4 to an inactive form of T3 called reverse T3 (rT3), and may be especially important during fetal development (Bianco, Salvatore et al. 2002).

SYMPTOMS OF HAVING A THYROID PROBLEM: WHAT PEOPLE MIGHT NOTICE

People can have certain *symptoms* (things they might notice that feels different than their usual state of health) or *signs* (physical exam or laboratory results findings) associated with disorders of the thyroid. Some of these symptoms might be due to an imbalance of thyroid hormone, i.e., too much or too little thyroid hormone, while other symptoms might be due to enlargement, tumor, or inflammation of the thyroid gland itself.

Enlargement of the thyroid is called a goiter. Occasionally only part of the thyroid is enlarged, but more often the entire gland is enlarged, sometimes even getting so large that it starts causing pressure on other organs in the neck such as the trachea (windpipe) or the esophagus (food pipe). Some goiters stick out and are visible upon looking at or examining the neck, whereas other goiters start slipping under the collarbone and can descend into the chest; this is called a substernal goiter. A very enlarge thyroid can cause a pressure sensation in the neck or cause trouble with the voice, breathing, or swallowing. Pain is very rare with thyroid enlargement.

Inflammatory conditions of the thyroid are generally called *thyroiditis.* While, in most people, the *immune system* is a guardian against infection and specialized cells attack bacteria and viruses, in thyroiditis, the immune system of the patient starts attacking the their own thyroid. This immune system gone awry can be specific to one organ, such as the thyroid, or can be part of a complex of other disorders called *autoimmune disease*. Most patients with thyroiditis at first might not notice any problems, but after a while the immune cells will attack and cause both structural and functional changes in the thyroid. In some cases, the immune cells make special proteins called *antibodies* that attack and destroy the thyroid tissue so the thyroid burns out and stops working normally. In other cases, the antibodies made have the opposite effect and stimulate the thyroid and cause overproduction of thyroid hormone.

Infection in the thyroid gland is quite rare, but when it happens, it is usually due to a virus. The thyroid gland will hurt or throb and can get enlarged. An infected thyroid gland can sometimes suddenly start leaking thyroid hormone, resulting in a burst of energy and thyroid hormone overactivity. Bacterial infections are very rare in the thyroid, but would usually lead to a collection of pus that may even need to be removed or drained out.

In *hyperthyroidism*, the thyroid is making too much thyroid hormone and people will notice signs of the imbalance of thyroid hormone. Too much thyroid hormone is not a good thing! The body and metabolism will be in overdrive and it won't be too long before the overactive cells will cause symptoms. The symptoms may be hard to notice at first, but if left untreated will eventually be very noticeable. Most commonly noticed symptoms include a racing heart, palpitations, diarrhea, weight loss, and a fine tremor. (See Table 2.2.)

In *hypothyroidism* the thyroid stops producing enough thyroid hormone and can eventually completely shut down. This is usually caused by a severe iodine deficiency or due to long standing autoimmune thyroiditis with burn out of the thyroid. People with hypothyroidism generally slow down, their cells are working but quite sluggishly, the person is barely getting by. The heart rate slows, the skin becomes dry and scaly, eyes can become puffy, energy levels are very low and the mind can become slow. In adults, even those with advanced symptoms of hypothyroidism can be fairly rapidly reversed by taking thyroid hormone prescribed by a physician. In young infants, however, if a low, functioning thyroid is not diagnosed expertly and quickly, there can be permanent problems with bone and brain development.

The thyroid can sometimes harbor small or large growths called *nodules*. Thyroid nodules are basically small lumps in the thyroid which can range in size from a small pea to the size of a golf ball or peach. Most of the nodules are benign growth and cause no symptoms, but if they do enlarge or become cancerous, thyroid nodules may press on the trachea or esophagus. Very large or cancerous nodules do need to be removed by expert surgeons. The most common kind of thyroid cancer is papillary thyroid cancer.

Table 2.2
Symptoms of Having Too Much Thyroid Hormone in Your Body

Clinical Presentation	
Hypothyroidism—Too Little	*Hyperthyroidism—Too Much*
As a newborn or infant:	Pounding of the heart (palpitations)
Cretinism, mental and growth retardation, short limbs	Increased heart rate
	Emotional instability
As an adult:	Tenseness, nervousness, irritability
In the short term:	Weight loss despite increased food intake
Tiredness and lethargy	Heat intolerance,
Cold intolerance	Decreased or absent menstrual flow
Constipation	Possibly enlarged thyroid gland
Poor appetite but gaining weight abnormal menstrual flow	Some eye changes including swollen or protruding eyes
Hair loss	Diarrhea
Brittle nails	Warm clammy skin
Dry coarse skin	Fine tremor
Hoarse voice	Excessive perspiration
In the long term if left untreated:	
Thickened features with swelling around eyes	
Swelling of hands and feet,	
Slow speech	
Sleepiness	
Slow mental function	
Muscle weakness	
Delayed reflexes	
Enlarged heart and heart failure	
Myxedema	
Low body temperature	

DOCTORS WHO WORK ON PATIENTS WITH THYROID DISEASES: SO MANY DOCTORS FOR ONE LITTLE GLAND—MUST MEAN IT'S IMPORTANT

Given the central importance of thyroid hormone on virtually all functions of the body, it should come as no surprise that any kind of doctor can detect a thyroid problem. Thyroid hormone imbalance can cause skin problems, mood disturbances, depression, infertility, pregnancy loss, heart rhythm problems, heart failure, and muscle weakness. . . . There are just too many to list. There are some doctors who routinely work only on diseases of the thyroid gland, these doctors are thyroid specialists.

Endocrinologists

Medical doctors who specialize in hormone producing *endocrine* organs such as the thyroid. They can order blood tests and imaging tests of the thyroid and can help diagnose these somewhat complex diseases.

Endocrine Surgeons

Surgeons who specialize in operations on the endocrine glands, including the thyroid, parathyroid, and pancreas. The commonest endocrine surgery operation is removal of the thyroid (thyroidectomy) and followed by parathyroid surgery (parathyroidectomy), followed by more rare operations on the adrenal gland (adrenalectomy). Endocrine surgeon have full training as general surgeons for five years followed by a one to two year fellowship which allows further specialization for removal of tumors from endocrine organs. Given the tight anatomic relations in the neck and the closeness of important structures and nerves, the extra expertise of these surgeons is needed if surgery on the thyroid gland is contemplated.

Ear/Nose and Throat Specialist or Otolaryngologist

Surgeons who specializes in the diagnosis and treatment of diseases of the ear, nose, and throat along with head and neck disorders. These doctors undergo surgical training composed of one year in general surgery and four years in otolaryngology—head and neck surgery. Since the thyroid is located near the throat, in some cases, these surgeons also specialize in surgery of the thyroid gland. Expertise of the surgeon is very important for good outcomes in thyroid surgery.

Radiologist

Medical doctors that utilize an array of imaging technologies (such as ultrasound, computed tomography (CT), nuclear medicine, positron emission tomography (PET), and magnetic resonance imaging (MRI) to diagnose or treat disease. Some radiologists specialize in imaging the thyroid gland in the body using ultrasound or special nuclear medicine tests. Sometimes their expertise is needed to use ultrasound guidance to help get a thin needle into the thyroid to withdraw cells for analysis under the microscope.

Pathologist/Cytologist

Pathologists are doctors who diagnose and characterize disease in living patients by examining biopsies, blood samples, or other bodily fluids. Additionally, pathologists interpret laboratory tests, making the majority of cancer diagnoses. In diagnosing thyroid cancers, pathologists examine tissue biopsies and fine needle aspiration samples under a microscope to analyze whether or not they are benign. Other pathologists specialize in genetic testing, which may help determine the most appropriate type of treatment. Pathologists also review results of tests ordered or performed by specialists, such as blood tests ordered by an endocrinologist. These doctors specialize in looking at organs, tissues, and cells under the microscope. Their expertise is often used to distinguish between benign and malignant (cancerous) growths in the thyroid.

Thyroid Researcher

Some doctors do not see patients but focus on research on diseases of the thyroid, looking for cures for both benign and malignant conditions. Thyroid research is a very broad and fascinating area of medicine both in the past and now. Many areas of interesting ongoing research involves thyroid physiology, effects of thyroid hormone on the gut, use of thyroid hormone for treatment of depression, and new ways to diagnose and combat thyroid cancer.

THYROID BLOOD TESTS: NOT TOO COMPLICATED

Doctors might measure certain blood factors to determine whether the thyroid gland is functioning and producing a normal level of thyroid hormone. Tests that measure the function of the thyroid gland are called *Thyroid Function Tests* (TFTs). When it is functioning normally, each person's thyroid tightly regulates the amount of thyroid hormone that is produced and released, making sure that there is always the proper amount for that individual. Naturally there is

Personal Notes: Learning from Experience
Comments from a Thyroid Pathologist

Dr. Yuri Nikiforov, a professor of pathology and director of the Division of Molecular Anatomic Pathology at the University of Pittsburgh Medical Center, has done extensive work on thyroid tumors and what makes them tick. He does research on how genetic and environmental damage drives the thyroid to develop. Originally from Belarus, he now lives in Pittsburgh with his wife and two children where he writes a personal note about how he managed to get where he is, what sparked his interest in the field of pathology, and a focus on the pathology of the thyroid gland.

I would lie to you if I say that I always wanted to be a thyroid pathologist, or even a pathologist. Remember that pathologists are physicians who look into a microscope to find how cells taken from a particular organ look and determine what is wrong with them. While in medical school, I enjoyed virtually all clinical specialties, but frequently had a feeling of some dissatisfaction at the end of the day. Becoming a doctor was difficult and it seemed impossible to come up with a definitive answer as to what the patient's problems and what were the causes of the symptoms the patient was experiencing.

I remember vividly my first day in a pathology lab. I looked into the microscope which had been set up by my professor and recognized a white blood cell that looked like it was trying to squeeze through a small hole in a blood vessel wall to get outside where I could see it was trying to join forces with other white blood cells gathered and busy attacking bacteria. These cells looked like troops fighting something. I asked my professor if this was just my imagination, but he smiled and replied that this is exactly how inflammation appears under the microscope and that this piece of tissue was taken from a lump on the patient's skin that was thought to be a cancer. When our professor examined it under the microscope, he noticed the same things I had and concluded that this happened to be just an inflammatory nodule caused by a skin infection. He was a pathologist but solved the puzzle and suggested that the patient be treated with antibiotics. I was amazed to realize that every human disease can be actually seen under the microscope as a remarkable constellation of colors and shapes formed by different cells and intercellular elements grouped in a specific patterns. Learning those patterns allowed diagnosing the disease with virtually absolute certainty. All you needed was just to learn all of those patterns. By the end of that day I pretty much knew that I wanted to be a pathologist.

Choosing thyroid pathology as my primary area of interest was influenced by an event that happened about 200 miles from my home in Belarus. On an unusually warm and sunny day in the spring of 1986, we found out that an accident happened at the Chernobyl nuclear power station. Initially details were scarce, but several days later we learned that an explosion at one of the nuclear reactors released a huge amount of radioactive materials and that many of these radioactive materials were specifically harmful to the thyroid gland, especially in children. It was a weird feeling to know that something harmful was surrounding us: something we could not see, smell, feel, or taste it. It was scary and surreal, almost like a science fiction movie. My two young brothers-in-law, who lived very close to Chernobyl, came to stay with us until it would be safe to return home. Early one morning, I took them to nearby government station to check the dose of radiation that they had received to their thyroid glands. Upon arrival we saw an enormous line of people, several thousands if not tens of thousands, mostly adults with kids. The line started at the bus station, snaked between the town's buildings, and went on for miles and miles. While I had been born many years after World War II, this looked like the evacuation stories my parents told about the war years when the German army was running through Belarus. Well, five or six hours later, completely exhausted, finally it was our turn. People in white coats were standing in front of a tent and quickly examining each child. The procedure was quite simple. A woman brought a tube-like device close to the neck of each of the boys, waited for a few seconds, and then shouted out "Below limit. Next!" This loud comment was apparently addressed to us and simultaneously to those next in line. The tone of her voice and her face transmitted a very clear message that no further clarification was going to be provided, no questions answered and we were to go on our merry way, grateful to have been "below the limit."

Several years later, I finished my pathology training and started working in a pediatric cancer center. There I started to notice an unusually high number of young children admitted for surgery due to thyroid cancer. In one year, we made more diagnoses of thyroid cancer in children than all my experienced pathology colleagues had made in the previous ten years. A little detective work showed that all these kids were from areas close to Chernobyl where the nuclear explosion had happened. My interest was piqued, what had radiation done to the thyroid glands of these children? By that point in my career, I had already a significant interest in thyroid gland pathology. I was puzzled by its complex yet logical microscopic structure, defined patterns of various diseases that affected the thyroid and by so many scientific questions about this gland that remained to be uncovered. From then on, I have been focusing on the pathology of the thyroid gland and my main scientific interest has been in understanding of how thyroid cancer develops after exposure to radiation. It has been a fascinating ride, frequently bumpy, at times frustrating, but never boring.

individual variation and one person might have more and another just a little less. In other words, there is just the right amount of thyroid hormone for each person, but everyone is within a particular range, which is called the *normal range*. The main thyroid function tests are listed below and they are rather simple and straightforward, though at first they may seem overwhelming. Thyroid hormone levels are measured by drawing a small tube of blood from patients and then analyzing the hormone levels in the serum and comparing it to levels seen in the general population. TFTs are most often measured by internists, though in some cases they may need the help of skilled thyroid specialists to interpret the results. Since many medications including birth control pills, estrogen compounds, blood pressure, and heart medicines may directly interfere with these blood tests and measurements, it is important to know which medications are being taken by the patient.

Thyroid Stimulating Hormone (TSH) Level

This is the most common first line blood test measured by doctors. This is a measure of how much signal is being sent out of the pituitary gland to help stimulate the thyroid gland. TSH measurements are very reliable but only work if there is a functional hypothalamic-pituitary axis and a working pituitary gland (that is the case in 99% of people). The pituitary gland constantly measures thyroid hormone levels in the blood of the patient, and if the pituitary gland senses that there is not enough thyroid hormone, the pituitary starts producing a special hormone called TSH. If the pituitary senses that there is too much thyroid hormone around, it will shut off TSH. The fine-tuned feedback system of the pituitary makes TSH the most sensitive indicator of an underactive or overactive thyroid, making this test the most commonly used test for detection of thyroid function abnormalities.

Low serum TSH levels: Indicates Hyperthyroidism (too much thyroid hormone)

High serum TSH levels: Indicates Hypothyroidism (too little thyroid hormone)

Normal TSH levels: Indicates a Euthyroid state (just the right amount of thyroid hormone) (see Figure 2.6)

T4 Level

Remember that T4 or L-thyroxine is the most common form of thyroid hormone produced in the thyroid gland. T4 is the hormone which ultimately helps regulate the body's metabolism. T4 levels will include T4 hormone that has been released from the thyroid and is circulating in the bloodstream. Some

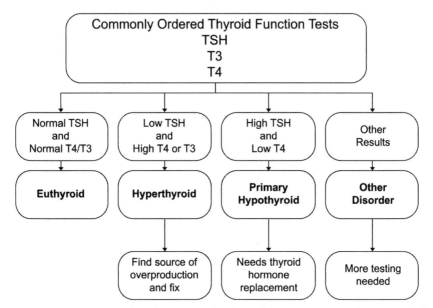

Figure 2.6   Common algorithms to use for thyroid function testing. (Drawn by Jeff Dixon after Dr. Sareh Parangi, MD)

of the T4 will be considered free T4, in other words it is not bound to any other proteins. Some of the T4 hormone will be bound to special carrier proteins. Both Free T4 and Total T4 levels are commonly measured by doctors, though Free T4 levels are more indicative of what is actually available for your body's cells to use as fuel. T4 hormone that is bound to other carrier proteins may be somewhat misleading especially if the carrier protein levels are too high such as during pregnancy or when taking birth control pills. Most doctors rely on the combination of two tests: free T4 levels and TSH to determine if a person is hyperthyroid or hypothyroid.

T3 Level

T4 hormone is processed into the biologic active form of thyroid hormone, T3. Most doctors will measure T3 levels to make sure enough of the biologically active T3 is around to meet the demands of the body. In some patients, plenty of T4 is made, but there is some kind of blockage in the next step of the processing. In these patients, there is plenty of T4 around, but TSH is still elevated signaling that the pituitary is sensing a lack of the active form of thyroid hormone and this is often the trigger for checking T3 levels. Some patients may not convert T4 to T3 because they are suffering from a severe systemic illness or recent surgery, others may be on powerful medications that can interfere with this conversion. One such medication is amiodarone, a heart medicine that practically shuts off conversion of T4 to T3.

Thyroglobulin

Thyroglobulin is a special protein that is coupled with iodine to make thyroid hormone inside the thyroid follicular cell. Some thyroglobulin is secreted into the bloodstream along with thyroid hormone levels, and everyone has a small amount in their bloodstream. If a person has too much thyroglobulin, it usually means there is either inflammation and leakage from the thyroid, the thyroid is very enlarged, or in some cases there is a thyroid cancer which is producing too much thyroglobulin. If the thyroglobulin level is elevated, an endocrinologist will try to determine the source of production by looking at your thyroid with scanning or ultrasound. If the source of the thyroglobulin is thyroid cancer, this means that the thyroglobulin is acting as a tumor marker and levels can be followed to look for cure of thyroid cancer after surgical removal of the thyroid and administration of radioactive iodine.

Anti-Thyroglobulin Antibodies

Some patients with autoimmune thyroid disease can produce special antibodies that attack thyroglobulin. It is important to know whether these antibodies are present in the blood stream because they make thyroglobulin measurements inaccurate. If a person has thyroglobulin antibodies, then thyroglobulin levels cannot be used to track tumor growth or look for thyroid cancer recurrence.

Anti-Thyroid Peroxidase Antibodies

Some patients with autoimmune thyroid disorders, especially those with auto-immune hypothyroidism, make strong antibodies that attack the special enzyme in the thyroid that processes iodine into thyroid hormone—thyroid peroxidase. High thyroid peroxidase antibody level usually predicts mild to moderate thyroid dysfunction and signal the fact that the thyroid may be on its way to burning out from *autoimmune hypothyroidism*.

Anti-TSH Receptor Antibodies

Some patients with autoimmune hyperthyroidism have special antibodies that constantly stimulate the thyroid by docking into the receptor for TSH and deceiving the thyroid into constant stimulation. This condition is called Graves' disease and these antibodies mimic the action of TSH which is normally regulated by the pituitary. These antibodies, however, have gone awry and result in constant stimulation of the thyroid and results in severe hyperthyroidism. Finding this particular antibody in high quantity in the serum is indicative of Graves' disease and on rare occasions, other forms of autoimmune thyroiditis.

IMAGING THE THYROID GLAND: HOW DOCTORS LOOK AT THE THYROID GLAND

Sometimes doctors need to get more information about the thyroid than is available by looking at blood tests. Remember that blood tests usually only show the level of thyroid hormone produced by the thyroid or the degree of inflammation in the thyroid. Blood tests cannot tell if there are congenital abnormalities in the development of the thyroid, or whether the thyroid is enlarged, or whether there are any abnormal lumps or "nodules" in the thyroid. Doctors use special X-ray machines and other ways to obtain images the thyroid gland. Some common methods look at the function of the thyroid and others look at the shape, size, and anatomy of the thyroid. This is a list of the commonly performed tests.

Ultrasonography

During ultrasonography, high-frequency sound waves are generated and used to view internal organs. The thyroid is a superficial organ in the neck and can be seen very well with ultrasound. Ultrasound is safe and non-invasive, does not use any radiation and is commonly used to detect nodules, cysts, and tumors of the thyroid. Ultrasound is almost always the first imaging test used in patients with thyroid problems because it is very good at looking at growths inside the thyroid gland.

Computed Axial Tomography (CAT Scan)

CAT scans use ionizing radiation to take precise thin cut pictures of the neck and thyroid gland which can then be put back together using computers. CAT scans are rarely used as a first tool in imaging the thyroid, since it is not very good at discerning differences between benign and cancerous growths in the thyroid. This test is very good at looking for enlarged thyroid goiters that have crept under the collarbone or for those with very large cancers which may be attached to other nearby organs.

An ultrasound image of the thyroid. The isthmus of the thyroid is seen as a thin gray strip on top of the trachea and the two lobes flank the trachea on each side. (iStock Photo)

Magnetic Resonance Imaging (MRI)

A common but relatively new radiologic imaging modality used to visualize detailed internal structure and limited function of the body. MRIs provide much greater contrast and details between the different soft tissues of the body than computed axial tomography (CAT) does for some body parts especially the brain. MRIs use no ionizing radiation but use a powerful magnetic field to align hydrogen atoms in water in the body. Radiofrequency fields are used to systematically alter the alignment of this magnetization, causing the hydrogen nuclei to produce a rotating magnetic field detectable by the scanner. This signal can be manipulated by additional magnetic fields to build up enough information to construct an image of the body. MRIs are also rarely used for those with thyroid problems. Some surgeons use this tool to look for lymph nodes which might be hiding cancer cells.

Radionuclide Scanning (Thyroid Scanning)

A form of nuclear medicine imaging in which radiopharmaceuticals are taken internally, for example intravenously or orally. Then, external detectors (gamma cameras) capture and form images from the radiation emitted by the radiopharmaceuticals. This process is unlike a diagnostic X-ray where external radiation is passed through the body to form an image. Diagnostic tests in nuclear medicine exploit the way that the body handles substances differently when there is disease or pathology present. The radionuclide introduced into the body is often chemically bound to a complex that acts characteristically within the body; this is commonly known as a tracer. In the presence of disease, a tracer will often be distributed around the body and/or processed differently. These tests generally look at the function of the thyroid gland by measuring how much iodine it can take up from the bloodstream in a set period of time.

^{123}I Scanning

^{123}I, a safe but radioactive tagged isotope of iodine, is injected into the bloodstream and accumulates in the thyroid. If one area of the thyroid is producing too much thyroid hormone, this area will show up as a "hot" spot or hot nodule in the pictures of the thyroid taken with a special gamma counter camera. ^{123}I scanning is only used to tell the function of the thyroid after blood tests have shown a suppressed TSH level thus indicating a nodule that may be producing too much thyroid hormone and thus suppressing the TSH level.

REFERENCES

Bianco, A. C., D. Salvatore, et al. (2002). "Biochemistry, cellular and molecular biology, and physiological roles of the iodothyronine selenodeiodinases." *Endocr Rev* **23**(1): 38–89.

Cohen, P. P. (1970). "Biochemical differentiation during amphibian metamorphosis." *Science* **168**(931): 533–43.

Crookes, P. F., and J. A. Recabaren (2001). "Injury to the superior laryngeal branch of the vagus during thyroidectomy: lesson or myth?" *Ann Surg* **233**(4): 588–93.

Heimeier, R. A., B. Das, et al. (2009). "The xenoestrogen bisphenol A inhibits postembryonic vertebrate development by antagonizing gene regulation by thyroid hormone." *Endocrinology* **150**(6): 2964–73.

3

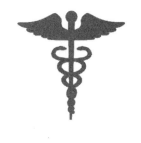

Conditions of the Thyroid That Can Affect People: What Can Go Wrong

HYPERTHYROIDISM: THE OVERACTIVE THYROID—TOO MUCH OF A GOOD THING

The terms hyperthyroidism and thyrotoxicosis are used interchangeably by many physicians, but actually refer to slightly different concepts. Hyperthyroidism (hyper is from the Greek word *huper* which means over) refers to overactivity of the thyroid gland, which leads to excess thyroid hormone production or peripheral conversion. Thyrotoxicosis (*thureos* is Greek for shield and *toxicos* is Greek for poison) refers to the clinical effects of excessive thyroid hormone, whether or not the problem is with the thyroid gland itself.

HYPERTHYROIDISM: THE BODY IN OVERDRIVE

Since thyroid hormone affects virtually every system in the body, people with hyperthyroidism develop a wide range of symptoms throughout their bodies (see Table 3.1). People may feel very anxious, easily irritable, and develop embarrassing tremors of their hands. People with hyperthyroidism may also note

Table 3.1
Symptoms of Hyperthyroidism

Anxiety

Restlessness

Irritability

Emotional instability

Fatigue

Muscle weakness or cramps

Increased appetite often with weight loss

Palpitations or an increased heart rate

Heat intolerance/increased sweating

Shortness of breath on exertion

Increased numbers of bowel movements or diarrhea

Tremor

Warm clammy skin

Decreased or absent menstrual flow

---

proximal muscle weakness that makes it difficult for them to lift heavier items or climb stairs. In severe instances of hyperthyroidism, people may require assistance to even stand up from a chair (Plummer's sign) due to weakness in their thigh muscles. Hyperthyroidism can also result in skin changes that cause people to have thinning hair and perspire more than normal. This may cause them to feel very uncomfortable in warmer climates and temperatures even when everyone else is comfortable. It can also affect the cardiovascular system and cause rapid or irregular heartbeats, which may become so severe as to cause a myocardial infarction (heart attack) or a cerebrovascular accident (stroke). People with hyperthyroidism also may note increased weight loss in spite of a normal or increased appetite with frequent, loose bowel movements and irregular menstrual periods. Finally, hyperthyroidism can cause decreased acuity in one's vision. Interestingly, elderly people with hyperthyroidism may not have many or any of the above symptoms. This lack of hyperthyroid symptoms in some patients is termed apathetic hyperthyroidism. Described originally in 1931 by Dr. Frank Lahey (one of the founders of the Lahey Clinic in Burlington, MA), this condition is characterized by blunted affect, lack of hyperkinetic motor activity, and slowed mentation in a patient who is thyrotoxic.

Table 3.2
Causes of Hyperthyroidism

Common Causes of Hyperthyroidism

Diffuse toxic goiter (Graves' disease)

Thyrotoxic phase of subacute thyroiditis

Toxic multinodular goiter (Plummer's disease)

Toxic adenoma

Less Common Causes of Hyperthyroidism

Iodide-induced thyrotoxicosis

Thyrotoxicosis factitia

Uncommon Causes of Hyperthyroidism

Pituitary tumors producing thyroid-stimulating hormone

Pituitary resistance to thyroid hormone

Excess human chorionic gonadotropin (molar pregnancy/choriocarcinoma)

Struma ovarii with thyrotoxicosis

Metastatic thyroid cancer

WHAT CAUSES HYPERTHYROIDISM?

People can develop hyperthyroidism for many reasons as shown in the Table 3.2.

DIFFUSE TOXIC GOITER: THE DISEASE WITH TOO MANY NAMES

The most common reason for hyperthyroidism is diffuse toxic goiter, which is known in the Western world as Graves' disease. It was described separately in medical literature by several physicians including Dr. Caleb Hillier Parry in 1825, by Dr. Robert James Graves in 1835, and by Dr. Carl A. von Basedow in 1840 (Hull 1998). In Europe, the term Basedow's disease is more commonly used than Graves' disease.

Regardless of the name, Graves' disease occurs when the body's natural defenses against infection (the immune system) stimulate the thyroid gland to produce too much thyroid hormone. No one is exactly sure what causes the body's immune system to do this to the thyroid gland, however, autoimmune thyroid disease has been linked to other autoimmune diseases that affect other organ systems including

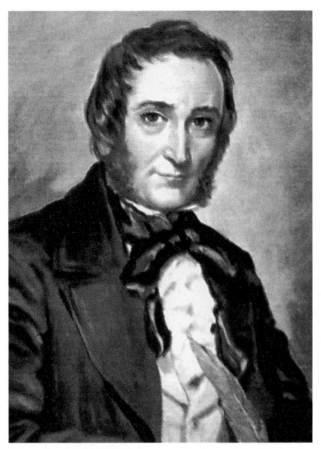

Dr. Robert James Graves (1796–1853) was an Irish surgeon. He was one of several physicians to describe the disease of diffuse toxic goiter. In the Western world, this disease still carries his name and is referred to as Graves' disease. (Armour Laboratories, Chicago/National Library of Medicine)

pernicious anemia, Sjogren's syndrome, Addison's disease, diabetes mellitus, myasthenia gravis, vitiligo, and primary biliary cirrhosis. People with Graves' disease typically have antibodies to thyroid peroxidase, thyroglobulin, and most-importantly to the thyroid stimulating hormone receptor. These antibodies lead to chronic stimulation of the thyroid gland, which leads to overproduction of thyroid hormone, and diffuse growth of the thyroid gland itself. These antibodies essentially trick the thyroid gland into thinking it constantly needs to produce thyroid hormone, even if there is already too much thyroid hormone around in the body.

Graves' disease typically affects young women between 20 and 50 years of age, although it has been reported to occur at any age in both men and women. The incidence of Graves' disease is approximately 3 percent of women and 0.3 percent of all men. Besides the previously mentioned symptoms of hyperthyroidism, people affected by Graves' disease often have problems with their eyes and skin.

The eye symptoms include problems with the eye orbit or eyeball itself as well as problems with the eyelids. Within the eye, antibodies in people with Graves' disease stimulate the production of glycosaminoglycans (large starch molecules) that attract water into the normally soft space behind the eyes. This movement of water increases the pressure behind the eye and the orbit, and causes the eye to bulge forward (*proptosis* or *exophthalmus*). Eventually, the pressure behind the eye can become so severe that there is damage to the blood and nerve supply to the eye leading to permanent blindness. Swelling from these glycosaminoglycans can also occur in the eyelids causing the eyelids to become puffy and retract. The combination of eyelid retraction and proptosis gives people with Graves' disease a characteristic constant surprised look or stare that can be socially awkward. The symptoms of eye disease associated with Graves' disease can be greatly exacerbated by the irritating effects of cigarette smoke.

Graves' disease can also rarely cause swelling of the skin called dermopathy. When this dermopathy occurs along a person's legs, it is called *pretibial myxedema*. The cause of the swelling associated with Graves' disease is believed to be similar to the eye swelling mentioned previously. Overstimulation of glycosaminoglycan production in the soft tissue spaces of the body causes water to move out of the bloodstream and into the skin, and since the skin around the shins is normally very tight, it often shows up there first.

Scintigraphy in Graves' disease demonstrates diffusely increase uptake (see Figure 3.1). The treatment of hyperthyroidism from Graves' disease includes medications to control the immediate symptoms of hyperthyroidism as well as decrease overall thyroid hormone synthesis. Many of the symptoms of hyperthyroidism including anxiety, heart palpitations, and tremor are due to an increased number of cellular receptors that respond to catecholamines or stress hormones. These receptors are called adrenergic receptors and are divided into two main groups, α and β receptors. A special class of medications called β-blockers, binds to β receptors and prevents their activation which helps reduce the symptoms of hyperthyroidism.

Another class of medications called thionamides can be used to control the amount of thyroid hormone synthesis. These medications are actively absorbed by the thyroid gland and prevent both the organification of iodine and the coupling of iodotyrosines into T3 or T4. Two popular thionamides in the United States are methimazole and propylthiouracil. Methimazole is generally preferred over propylthiouracil as it remains in the body longer and therefore only needs to be taken once a day. Both medications should be used with great caution in pregnant patients.

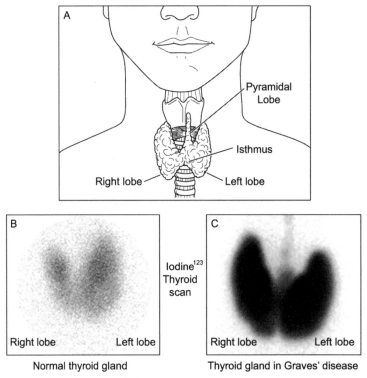

Figure 3.1   Thyroid radionuclide scanning in a patient with hyperthyroidism reveals diffuse enlargment of the thyroid with overproduction of thyroid hormone in the entire thyroid consistent with Graves' disease. (Drawn by Jeff Dixon after Dr. Sareh Parangi, MD)

Both β-blockers and thionamides are temporary treatments of hyperthyroidism only. Permanent forms of treatment include radioactive iodine and/or surgery which are discussed in later chapters.

SUBACUTE THYROIDITIS: INFLAMMATION IN THE THYROID

Subacute thyroiditis is the second most common cause of hyperthyroidism. It occurs when the body's own immune system attacks the thyroid and causes release of too much thyroid hormone, sometimes due to an infection in the thyroid and other times due to a particular medication the person might be taking.

Subacute granulomatous thyroiditis (also known as *de Quervain's* thyroiditis), is probably caused by infection of the thyroid gland with viral particles. People with this form of subacute thyroiditis may present with high fever, malaise (feeling unwell), myalgia (joint pains), fatigue, and severe neck pain that may limit their

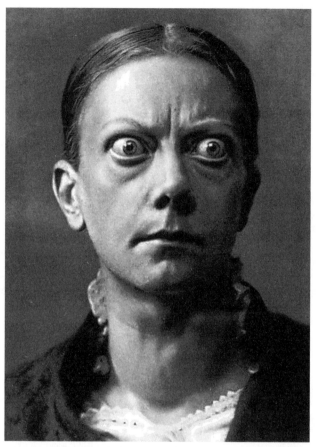

A patient with advanced signs of hyperthyroidism including retraction of the eyelids, bulging of the eyes, a large swollen thyroid, and prominent neck veins. The illustration appeared in Byrom Bramwell's *Atlas of Clinical Medicine* (1893). (National Library of Medicine)

ability to swallow. This pain typically starts in the lower neck and can then radiate to the jaw or ear on that side. Thyroid hormone levels are often extremely elevated, resulting in marked signs and symptoms of thyrotoxicosis mentioned previously. Patients with subacute granulomatous thyroiditis may have a genetic predisposition or sensitivity to various virus particles that have been implicated with this thyroid condition including influenza, adenovirus, mumps, and coxsackievirus. This infection ultimately results in destruction of the thyroid gland and release of thyroid hormone from the damaged thyroid cells. It is unclear whether the destructive thyroiditis is caused by direct viral infection of the gland

One More Thing to Know: Now That's Interesting
Thyroid Physiology: Lessons from the White House

U.S. President George H. W. Bush had not been looking quite right to his secretary for a couple of weeks in the spring of 1991. He had trouble signing documents. He was getting weighed daily and despite his voracious appetite, he was losing weight. On May 4, 1991, the president felt faint while running and his personal physician Dr. Nash evaluated him. He had an irregular heart beat. He was in atrial fibrillation and after 24 hours, his thyroid function tests revealed a markedly decreased TSH. His thyroid was overactive, and he was diagnosed with Grave's disease. He had none of the eye symptoms common with Graves' disease, but the condition was significant enough that he had to be treated with radioactive iodine to render his thyroid non functional.

It is interesting that President Bush's wife, First Lady Barbara Bush also suffered from Graves' disease since 1989. The fact that the couple had the same disease is probably coincidental and is not surprising since over one million Americans have this autoimmune disease named after the nineteenth-century physician Dr. Robert Graves who first reported it. In Graves' disease the eye problems can occur before or after the thyroid symptoms. The severity of the eye problems does not necessarily parallel the degree of overactivity of the thyroid gland. Some people with Graves' disease suffer more from the thyroid condition, and some suffer more from the eye problems.

She, however, did have significant eye disease associated with her condition and had eye protrusion (exopthalmus) which can be appreciated in many of her portraits. Mrs. Bush was treated with both medications and dose of radioactive iodine, after which she was advised not to embrace her grandchildren for a few weeks as a precaution. Her eye problems did not improve even though she was no longer hyperthyroid, she was treated ultimately with radiation beams to her eyes in 1990.

Untreated Graves' disease can even be fatal, so it is lucky for the United States that the condition was diagnosed early and treated. President Bush's episode of hyperthyroidism led to some newspaper articles such as "Desert Storm or Thyroid Storm" looking at the role of his overactive thyroid in his decision making process. Graves' disease, like other autoimmune conditions, is often thought to come on during times of stress, and certainly with the first Gulf War. The year of 1991 was a stressful year for the president because of the remarkable coincidence of two cases of auto-immune disease in one household, three if you consider their dog Millie was also diagnosed with Lupus, the Secret Service tested the water in the White House, at Camp David, at the vice president's residence, and at Walker's Point (Bush's home in Maine) for lithium and iodine, two substances "known to cause thyroid problems" (Altman 1991; James F. Toole 2001).

or by the host's response to the viral infection. It is important to remember that granulomatous thyroiditis is not an autoimmune disease of the thyroid.

In *lymphocytic thyroiditis*, which is often painless, something triggers the body's immune system to attack the thyroid, often due to medications the person might be on for other conditions or due to pregnancy. Common medications used to treat heart disease, cancer, or psychiatric disorders can trigger inflammation in the thyroid. *Amiodarone* is a drug used to control arrhythmias of the heart and almost 30 percent of its weight is iodine. Therefore, people who have to take amiodarone for their heart conditions are getting excessive amounts of iodine everyday, which results in a destructive inflammatory condition of the thyroid and the release of too much thyroid hormone. This form of thyroiditis is more common in men, likely due to the higher prevalence of amiodarone therapy in men and typically occurs after more than two years of amiodarone therapy. Another medication that may stimulate lymphocytic thyroiditis is *interferon-alpha* which is used for the treatment of many different types of human cancers and also viral diseases such as hepatitis. Approximately five percent of patients on interferon-alpha therapy may develop lymphocytic thyroiditis after about three months of treatment for reasons that are not completely understood. Symptoms of hyperthyroidism are typically very mild so this form of thyroiditis is usually diagnosed on the basis of abnormal test results as opposed to clinical signs and symptoms. Another medication that may cause lymphocytic thyroiditis is *lithium*. Lithium is a metal that is typically used in the treatment of psychiatric disorders such as bipolar disease. Lithium directly inhibits the release of thyroid hormone and can cause either subclinical or clinical hypothyroidism and thyroid goiter. However, lithium therapy can also cause lymphocytic thyroiditis possibly due to either increased thyroid antibody production or a direct toxic effect of lithium on the thyroid gland. Lymphocytic thyroiditis from lithium may also occur up to five months following discontinuation of lithium therapy.

The last form of subacute thyroiditis occurs after pregnancy so it is aptly termed *subacute postpartum thyroiditis* (after giving birth). This condition is likely autoimmune in nature and in iodine-sufficient countries, such as the United States, tends to occur in approximately five to eight percent of pregnant women. These women will often present to their physician one to six months postpartum with painless thyroid enlargement and elevated thyroid hormone levels. They may report a sudden burst of energy, lack of sleep, nervousness, fatigue, and easy weight loss, which unfortunately is difficult to differentiate from the normal changes in physiology that occur after pregnancy. Women who smoked cigarettes or have positive test results for thyroid auto-antibodies either before their pregnancy or during the third trimester are at much higher risk of developing postpartum thyroiditis. Also, women who have subacute postpartum thyroiditis are likely to have additional episodes following subsequent pregnancies.

The good news is that subacute thyroiditis is almost always a self-limiting thyroid condition that will improve with supportive care only. People who have subacute granulomatous thyroiditis may require nonsteroidal anti-inflammatory medications (such as ibuprofen or naproxen) to reduce neck pain symptoms. In rare instances, narcotics pain medicine and glucocorticoid steroids may be required to achieve adequate pain control for people experiencing extreme neck pain. People with severe symptoms of hyperthyroidism from subacute thyroiditis may require a medication called ipodate (iopanoic acid or Gastrografin), to inhibit the peripheral conversion of T4 to T3.

TOXIC NODULAR GOITER: NOT AS BAD AS IT SOUNDS

Toxic nodular goiter is also known as Plummer's disease, named after the physician Dr. Henry Stanley Plummer who originally described this thyroid disease in 1913. Toxic nodular goiter is the second most common cause of hyperthyroidism in the United States (15–30%) and represents a spectrum of disease that includes a single hyperfunctioning adenoma (toxic adenoma) in an otherwise normal thyroid gland, to multiple hyperfunctioning adenomas in a multinodular enlarged thyroid (toxic multinodular goiter). Hyperthyroidism typically occurs when at least a single nodule is greater than 2.5 cm in diameter, and often presents in elderly people with a long history of thyroid goiter. The excess production of thyroid hormone is typically gradual and it may take many years for symptoms to develop. Scintigraphy of a thyroid gland with toxic nodular disease demonstrates areas of increased uptake, which corresponds to the areas of the gland that are hyperfunctioning. The areas of decreased uptake on scintigraphy represent normal suppressed thyroid tissue.

The cause of thyroid toxic nodular disease is not completely understood, but it is believed that overall iodine deficiency leads to low levels of thyroid hormone, which subsequently stimulates thyroid cell growth (hyperplasia). The increased rate of thyroid cell division predisposes single cells to genetic mutations of the TSH receptor. Activation of this receptor may stimulate further copies of these thyroid cells with a mutated TSH receptor in a process called clonal proliferation. These clones are ultimately organized into thyroid nodules.

IODINE INDUCED THYROTOXICOSIS: MUCH TOO MUCH

Taking in food or medications with too much iodine can cause hyperthyroidism, especially if a person's thyroid was already under constant TSH stimulation. For example, Dr. Basedow noted that giving someone iodine when they previously had baseline iodine deficiency can trigger severe episodes of hyperthyroidism. This phenomenon is called the Jod-Basedow phenomenon (*Jod* means iodine in German).

Laboratory evaluation in a person who has hyperthyroidism from excessive iodine, typically demonstrates increased levels of plasma thyroglobulin, iodine, and thyroid hormone levels. Discontinuation of the offending agent is the treatment of choice and symptomatic therapy with a beta-blocker medication may be helpful.

THYROTOXICOSIS FACTITIA: THE TRUTH ALWAYS COMES OUT

Another less common cause of hyperthyroidism is thyrotoxicosis factitia. It is hyperthyroidism that is induced intentionally or accidentally by short or long-term ingestion of thyroid hormone. Sometimes this disorder is caused by accidental ingestion. For example, a child reaches into his mother's purse and takes her thyroid medication because he thought it was candy. Another method of accidental ingestion has been termed "hamburger" thyrotoxicosis, which occurs if a cow's thyroid gland is accidentally introduced into ground beef at a meat preparation facility. Even if the thyroid-contaminated beef is subsequently cooked at high temperatures, eating it can result in small outbreaks of hyperthyroidism. Thyrotoxicosis factitia can also refer to people who have a psychiatric disorder that compels them to surreptitiously use thyroid hormone. These people may have a desire to hurt themselves or may want to induce mild hyperthyroidism and weight loss. In all of these situations, people with thyrotoxicosis factitia have elevated levels of thyroid hormone and suppressed concentrations of TSH. This leads to shrinkage of the thyroid gland, which differentiates thyrotoxicosis factitia from other forms of hyperthyroidism that usually have an enlarged thyroid gland. The treatment of thyrotoxicosis factitia is essentially symptomatic and discontinuation of the thyroid hormone. For acute accidental ingestions, it is recommended to induce emesis and wash out of the stomach to prevent continued absorption of the thyroid hormone. Symptoms of hyperthyroidism can be controlled with beta-blocking agents, barbiturates, digoxin, hydrocortisone, and cooling blankets. In life-threatening situations, plasmapheresis or filtering of the blood could be used, although this will only remove about 25 to 30 percent of the total ingested dose. Finally, as mentioned previously, sodium ipodate (Orografin or Gastrografin), reduces peripheral tissue uptake of thyroid hormones and helps to relieve many of the symptoms of hyperthyroidism in the short-term.

NOT SO COMMON CAUSES OF HYPERTHYROIDISM: NOT YOUR EVERYDAY FARE

Uncommon causes of hyperthyroidism include secondary hyperthyroidism, human chorionicgonadotropin-secreting tumors (hCG), struma ovarii with thyrotoxicosis, and metastatic thyroid cancer.

SECONDARY HYPERTHYROIDISM

Secondary hyperthyroidism is a very rare phenomenon that occurs either from a small benign tumor growing in the pituitary gland (*pituitary adenoma*) or from pituitary resistance to thyroid hormone. In the first instance, a small tumor "pushes" onto the pituitary gland causing the uncontrolled release of all pituitary hormones including thyroid stimulating hormone (TSH), growth hormone, prolactin, follicle-stimulating hormone, leutinizing hormone, adrenocorticotropic hormone, oxytocin, and vasopressin. Therefore, a person with hyperthyroidism from a pituitary adenoma typically has signs of hyperthyroidism mixed with other hormonal imbalances including uncontrolled growth, hair production, or lactation (milk expressed from mammary tissue). Laboratory studies would demonstrate elevated or normal TSH levels in the face of high T3 and T4, which indicates inappropriate secretion of TSH by the pituitary gland. It is also possible that the pituitary adenoma itself is producing thyroid stimulating hormone. A magnetic resonance imaging (MRI) scan of the head may reveal the small tumor in the pituitary gland. The treatment would be to remove the mass through the back of the nose, which is called *transsphenoidal surgical resection.*

Another cause of secondary hyperthyroidism is *pituitary resistance* to thyroid hormone, specifically resistance to thyroxine. This disease is also very rare and can occur as a spontaneous mutation or can be inherited as an autosomal dominant trait from a person's parents. Because the pituitary gland is not responsive to thyroxine, the feedback to the furnace fails (see Chapter 2). Therefore, the levels of TSH are high and thyroid hormones continue to be secreted. Pituitary resistance to thyroid hormone can be distinguished from a pituitary adenoma by a thyroid releasing hormone (TRH) stimulation test. Patients with resistance to thyroid hormone have a normal rise in TSH in response to TRH administration. In contrast, patients with pituitary tumors have a high baseline TSH but little or no response to TRH stimulation. Interestingly, attention deficit hyperactivity disorder has been associated with the syndrome of pituitary resistance to thyroid hormone. Treatment for pituitary resistance to thyroxine is very difficult to treat. The pituitary may respond to inhibition with dopamine agonists or high levels of T3. Treatment of the symptoms of hyperthyroidism may also be helpful including beta-blockers and anti-thyroid medications.

Tumors That Can Lead to Thyrotoxicosis

Struma ovarii is a tumor in the ovary called a teratoma (pronounced tear–a–toe–mah) and contains more than 50 percent thyroid tissue. This type of tumor and usually but not always found in the ovary. It is very rare (only 3% of all ovarian teratomas) and is composed of embryonic germ cells or precursor cells that can differentiate into thyroid cells and then secrete thyroid hormone independent of the normal "furnace" feedback mechanisms. People with struma ovarii typically present with abdominal or lower pelvic pain and only incidentally are found to have an ovarian tumor. Presentation of this disease can occur at any age, but is most common in the fifth to sixth decade of life. Clinical hyperthyroidism only develops in five to ten percent of all patients with struma ovarii. When the tumor is removed surgically, the thyroid tissue inside the teratoma is almost always benign (99.7–99.9% of the time). In extremely rare circumstances, a thyroid carcinoma (papillary, follicular variant of papillary, or follicular) has been found inside a struma ovarii.

Another type of tumor that can lead to thyrotoxicosis are *hydatidiform moles* and *choriocarcinomas*. Hydatidiform moles are products of an abnormal pregnancy wherein a non-viable, fertilized egg implants in the uterus, and thereby converts normal pregnancy processes into pathological ones. No identifiable embryonic or fetal tissues arise when an empty egg with no nucleus is fertilized by one (or occasionally two) normal sperm. Human chorionic gonadotropin (hCG) is a glycoprotein that is synthesized by the placenta during pregnancy and can directly bind to the TSH receptors on the thyroid gland and stimulate thyroid hormone release. This not typically a problem during pregnancy given the small amounts of hCG normally produced. However, hydatidiform mole and choriocarcinomas can secrete large amounts of hCG which can result in thyrotoxicosis. In some patients, these hCG levels may attain several-fold the peak levels of normal pregnancy. The usual presentation of a hydatidiform mole is abnormal vaginal bleeding during pregnancy with very high hCG levels in the bloodstream. When a hydatidiform mole is discovered, the treatment is to remove it in the operating room through the vagina. The treatment of choriocarcinomas, on the other hand, requires specialized medical treatment.

Thyroid cancer that has metastasized to distant places in the body can rarely lead to excessive thyroid hormone production. This is discussed in detail in Chapter 5.

HYPOTHYROIDISM

Hypothyroidism (hypo in Latin means low) is the most common thyroid disorder in the world and is thought to affect over ten million people in the United States alone. It is characterized by the insufficient production of thyroid hormone. The 1999–2002 National Health and Nutrition Examination Survey studied 4,392 Americans and found a higher incidence of hypothyroidism in Caucasians and Mexican-Americans (5.1%) compared to African-Americans (1.7%). There are several common causes of hypothyroidism. The incidence of hypothyroidism increases as a person becomes older and is most common after the age of sixty.

WHAT DOES HYPOTHYROIDISM FEEL LIKE?
RUNNING ON EMPTY

Since thyroid hormone plays an important role in regulating our normal metabolism, symptoms of hypothyroidism are related to a "slowing down" of metabolic processes in every system of the human body. Many of the symptoms of hypothyroidism are vague and may be mistakenly attributed to normal aging. The symptoms typically worsen as the degree of hypothyroidism increases over time.

For example, a person with hypothyroidism may feel sluggish, feel mentally depressed, and find it difficult to concentrate with a general slowing of speech and natural muscle reflexes. Hypothyroidism can make a person feel fatigued easily; experience muscle cramps, modest gain in body weight (usually 10–15 pounds), increased serum cholesterol levels, or difficulty losing weight, and feel cold when everyone else is comfortable. A person with hypothyroidism may also have skin changes such as decreased sweating, puffiness around the eyes, and dry, flaky, or thick skin. The hair may become coarse and thin, with loss of eyebrows and development of brittle finger and toenails. Insufficient amounts of thyroid hormone can also lead to decreased functioning of the heart and lungs, which may lead to increasing shortness of breath with minimal exertion, high blood pressure (hypertension), or even heart failure. Hypothyroidism can even affect a person's gastrointestinal tract causing a decrease in normal peristaltic (means wave-like) motions that can lead to severe constipation. Women with hypothyroidism may have absent or infrequent menstrual cycles which can make it difficult to become pregnant. Each person is unique so people living with hypothyroidism may have none, some, or all of these symptoms. In people with severe cases of untreated hypothyroidism, physiological stress to the body such as injuries, infections, or even exposure to cold temperatures can trigger a life-threatening condition called *myxedema coma*.

Myxedema coma is a true endocrine emergency, but its name is somewhat misleading as many people with this disorder are not, in fact, in a coma. The major clinical hallmarks of myxedema coma include poor mentation, hypothermia, hemodynamic instability, lethargy, respiratory acidosis that all eventually may progress to coma, and then ultimately death, if untreated. Although all age groups can be affected, elderly women during the winter months are more prone to myxedema coma. Laboratory studies demonstrate decreased T4 and T3 levels and elevated TSH level. Initially, death rates from myxedema coma were very high in the range of 60 to 70 percent. However, numerous advances in critical care technologies have reduced the mortality rates to 20 to 25 percent. The mainstay of therapy for people with myxedema consists of thyroid hormone replacement, supportive measures aimed at cardiovascular, respiratory, and neurologic systems, and managing any coexisting problems especially infections.

The causes of hypothyroidism can be grouped into primary hypothyroidism, secondary hypothyroidism, and tertiary hypothyroidism.

PRIMARY HYPOTHYROIDISM: IT'S ALL THE THYROID'S FAULT

Primary hypothyroidism is when the cause of hypothyroidism is from the thyroid gland itself. This is the most common reason for hypothyroidism (95%) and may be due to inflammation of the thyroid gland, medications, or from medical treatments. Past or currently on-going inflammation of thyroid gland may damage or destroy normal thyroid cells. This process ultimately leaves a person with too little thyroid tissue to produce enough thyroid hormone for their body.

The most common cause of thyroid inflammation is an inherited condition called *Hashimoto's thyroiditis* (see sidebar on Dr. Hakaru Hashimoto). This inflammation is autoimmune mediated meaning that a person's body incorrectly views the thyroid gland as an intruder and inappropriately attacks and destroys normal thyroid cells. Chronic destruction of thyroid cells occurs at a pace that is faster than the body can replace them, leaving just a few working thyroid cells in a desert of scar tissue. The types of antibodies that are found in people with Hashimoto's thyroiditis include antimicrosomal, antithyroid peroxidase (anti-TPO), and antithyroglobulin antibodies. These antibodies may not be present early in the disease process and usually disappear over time.

As mentioned previously, people with subacute thyroiditis may initially present with hyperthyroidism that may eventually leads to a short period of hypothyroidism as the thyroid gland heals from the autoimmune-mediated attack.

DRUG-INDUCED HYPOTHYROIDISM:
THE INNOCENT BYSTANDER

Some medications can cause hypothyroidism. In some cases, this is intentional and the medications are prescribed to cause the thyroid hormone to decrease or stop producing thyroid hormone. In other case, medications given for other diseases can lead to effects on the production of thyroid hormone.

One group of medications can have some puzzling effects: medications that contain the mineral iodine. Some of these medications contain large amounts of iodine such as Amiodarone (Cordarone) and potassium iodide (SSKI, Pima, and Lugol's solution). Taking a large dose of these medications can suppress normal

**Historical Perspectives: How One Person Can Make a Difference
Dr. Hashimoto's Role in Discovering the Most Common
Reason for Hypothyroidism**

Dr. Hakaru Hashimoto (1881–1934) was born on May 5, 1,881, in the village of Midau, Nishi-tsuge, in the Mie Prefecture. He was the third son in a long ancestral line of physicians, so it was no surprise when he chose to pursue a career in medicine and graduated from Kyushu Imperial University medical school in 1907.

Between 1908 and 1912, Dr. Hashimoto took an interest in thyroid tissue while working in a surgical department. He extracted thyroid tissue samples from four middle-aged women with goiters and noted that unlike a typical goiter, these thyroid samples had a preponderance of lymphoid tissue. Specifically, Dr. Hashimoto noted the formation of lymphoid follicles, the marked changes in the thyroid epithelial cells, the extensive formation of new connective tissue and the diffuse round cell infiltration. He named these changes "struma lymphomatosa" and decided to publish his observations in a German surgical journal named *Archiv Fur Klinishe Chirurgie*, as he thought this would make more of an international impact than an article in Japanese. This article was approximately 30 pages long with five figures and was his only publication on the thyroid gland. However, his observations of lymphocytic thyroiditis went largely unnoticed in the English-speaking world, despite his effort.

Dr. Hashimoto then traveled to Germany to study pathology under Professor Eduard Kaufmann at Goettingen University. However, he was forced to return to Kyusyu University with the start of World War I. A short time later, Dr. Hashimoto returned to his birthplace to take over the family medical practice because his family needed financial support. He soon became very popular among the local communities for his great international knowledge of medicine as well as his compassion towards the sick. Unfortunately, at the age of 52, Dr. Hashimoto became infected with typhoid fever during one of his house calls and subsequently died on Jan. 9, 1934.

Shortly after his death, Dr. Allen Graham, a surgeon from Cleveland, Ohio, "rediscovered" and popularized Dr. Hashimoto's observations. Soon after, Hashimoto began to be mentioned in thyroid surgery textbooks and his name was routinely attached to the disease in America. To honor, Dr. Hashimoto's accomplishments, the Japan Thyroid Association chose his picture as their new logo when the group was founded in 1958 (Sawin 2002; Takami, Miyabe et al. 2008).

thyroid function and lead to hypothyroidism. This result is counter-intuitive since one would think that extra iodine would cause hyperthyroidism, right? Sudden ingestion of very large amounts of iodine can actually result in hypothyroidism through a physiological mechanism originally theorized by Drs. Jan Wolff and Israel Lyon Chaikoff in 1948. Although the exact mechanism for the Wolff-Chaikoff effect is still not clear even after all of these years, it clearly prevents the release of massive amounts of thyroid hormone when the human body is given large dosages of iodine. Normal organification of iodide typically resumes in several days through an "escape" form the Wolff-Chaikoff anti-organification effect. However, some individuals may develop a permanent state of hypothyroidism for unclear reasons, especially if they do not have a normal thyroid gland at baseline. Lithium (Eskalith and Lithobid) is a common medication used to treat bipolar and other psychiatric conditions can also lead to hypothyroidism after a period of hyperthyroidism due to thyroid "burnout." As mentioned previously, lithium directly blocks the production of thyroid hormone. Finally, medications used to treat hyperthyroidism (see previous section) such as methimazole (Tapazole) and propylthiouracil (PTU), may ultimately lead to hypothyroidism. All of the symptoms of hypothyroidism should resolve after the causative medication is stopped.

SECONDARY AND TERTIARY HYPOTHYROIDISM: IT'S NOT THE THYROID'S FAULT

Secondary hypothyroidism is when a person's pituitary gland is diseased or injured which causes too little thyroid stimulating hormone (TSH) to be produced. Without the signal to produce more thyroid hormone, the thyroid gland becomes quiescent and the person develops hypothyroidism. This cause of hypothyroidism is very rare and is typically associated with other hormonal imbalances from lack of pituitary stimulation to other endocrine organs.

Tertiary hypothyroidism is when there is damage to a person's hypothalamus that prevents the release of thyroid releasing hormone. This prevents the thyroid furnace (see Chapter 2) from receiving any signal to start and may be due to a mass growing in the hypothalamus or brain trauma. The diagnosis and treatment of hypothyroidism relies on the fact that exogenous thyroid releasing hormone corrects the person's thyroid hormone levels.

TREATMENT OF HYPOTHYROIDISM—BRINGING THINGS BACK INTO BALANCE

The goals for the treatment of hypothyroidism are to bring the body back into balance with just the right amount of thyroid hormone and thyroid stimulating hormone. Initially in the 1950s, thyroid hormone replacement was given in the form of "thyroid extract" obtaining by grinding and processing thyroids obtained from animals. The problem with this method was that the concentration of thyroid hormone varied widely from one batch of medications to the other. Nowadays, synthetic thyroid hormone (Synthroid, Levoxyl, Levothyroid, Unithroid, and levothyroxine) is given to people suffering from hypothyroidism. The actual dosage of synthetic thyroid hormone is very small and is usually around 1.6 micrograms per kilogram of body weight per day. Elderly people with hypothyroidism are usually started slowly on replacement synthetic thyroid hormone as too much thyroid hormone can cause arrhythmias or even a heart attack (myocardial infarction).

As mentioned previously (in Chapter 2), the most active form of thyroid hormone is triiodothyronine (T3), so why do doctors give patients with hypothyroidism thyroxine (T4) instead of T3? The answer lies in the fact that T3 is metabolized so quickly that a person with hypothyroidism would have to take it several times a day. In addition, T3 is very active and can lead to a "boost" of thyroid hormone which can lead to feeling like the person has had too much coffee. Thyroxine is normally taken only once a day and is converted in the body to T3.

After therapy with thyroid hormone has started, it takes a few weeks for the thyroid stimulating hormone and thyroid hormone levels to start normalizing. Symptoms of hypothyroidism slowly resolve over a period of several weeks to months. Periodic measurements of thyroid stimulating hormone and thyroid hormone levels are sometimes needed as the dosage of synthetic thyroid hormone that a person needs fluctuates depending on age, weight, and other diseases or medications.

THYROID DISEASE IN INFANTS AND CHILDREN

Though thyroid disease in infants and children is rare, they have been studied intently since getting the right balance of thyroid hormone is extremely important for both brain and body development. Infants and children can have either hypothyroidism or hyperthyroidism for a variety of reasons. The causes for hypothyroidism in infants and children can be loosely divided into congenital (born with the condition) versus acquired hypothyroidism (happens during childhood due to a disease process).

HYPOTHYROIDISM IN CHILDREN: BETTER DIAGNOSE IT PRONTO!

Approximately 75 percent of the time, congenital hypothyroidism is due to defective thyroid gland development or *dysgenesis*. There is a spectrum of severity with thyroid dysgenesis that can be as minor as incomplete formation of the thyroid with partial function remaining (*hypoplasia*) to lack of any thyroid tissue and therefore no thyroid function at all (*agenesis*). Laboratory testing and imaging can determine the degree of thyroid function and amount of dysgenesis. Another form of congenital hypothyroidism is *familial thyroid dyshormonogenesis*, which can occur as a result of any number of rare autosomal recessive defects in thyroid hormone synthesis, secretion, or uptake. These defects can occur anywhere along the complex mechanism of action of thyroid hormone including defects in: TSH receptors, organification of iodine, coupling of iodotyrosines, thyroglobulin synthesis or proteolysis, or the release of T3 and T4 into the body's circulatory system. People with congenital hypothyroidism may also have partial peripheral resistance to thyroid hormone, which means that higher amounts of thyroid hormone are needed to achieve the same effect. Finally, secondary and tertiary hypothyroidism can also occur in infants and children from either congenital or acquired problems with the hypothalamic-pituitary axis.

Temporary congenital hypothyroidism is typically acquired from the newborn's mother while the newborn is still in the mother's womb. Maternal exposure to large amounts of iodine, anti-thyroid medications, or goitrogens may all temporarily suppress the newborn's thyroid gland. These effects may be temporary depending on when the fetus was exposed to the external agents. In mothers with autoimmune thyroiditis, anti-thyroid antibodies from the mother can travel across the placenta to the developing fetus. These antibodies block the TSH receptors on the fetal thyroid gland resulting in hypothyroidism at birth. The newborn will likely require supplementation of thyroid hormone until the antibodies are completely destroyed in about two to three months after birth.

Similar to adults, acquired hypothyroidism in infants and children is typically due to a chronic lymphocytic thyroiditis conditions such as autoimmune thyroiditis or Hashimoto's disease. Subacute thyroiditis is rare in children, but presents in a similar fashion as in adults and rarely requires treatment. Lastly, environmental factors such as iodine deficiency, exposure to certain types of medications, and massive irradiation (consider the Chernobyl nuclear melt-down level of radiation) may all lead to hypothyroidism in children.

HYPERTHYROIDISM IN CHILDREN: WATCH OUT FOR THOSE ANTIBODIES AGAIN

Unlike hypothyroidism, hyperthyroidism is a relatively rare condition in children. Graves' disease causes 95 percent of all cases of childhood hyperthyroidism. The presentation, diagnosis, and treatment of childhood Graves' disease is virtually identical to the adult form of Graves' disease.

Neonatal Graves' disease, on the other hand, is very different from adult Graves' disease and accounts for less than one percent of all cases of hyperthyroidism in pediatric patients. Virtually all babies with Graves' disease have a maternal history of Graves' disease, either during the pregnancy or at some time in the past. Neonatal Graves' disease is caused by the transplacental passage of thyroid stimulating antibodies from the mother to the baby. These antibodies stimulate the baby's thyroid gland as well causing in-utero symptoms of hyperthyroidism and diffuse goiter formation. These antibodies should be removed from the baby's system by the time the baby is three to four months of age. Because maternal antibodies cause neonatal Graves' disease, it is self-limited and the symptoms of hyperthyroidism typically resolve by the time the child is three to four months of age.

If the baby's mother is taking antithyroid medications, infants with neonatal Graves' disease are usually born asymptomatic. Signs and symptoms may become manifest when antithyroid medications that have crossed the placenta are cleared from the infant's bloodstream. Complications of neonatal Graves' disease include congestive heart failure, airway compression from the large goiter, craniosynostosis (early closure of skull bones), and developmental delay.

Another cause of hyperthyroidism that is unique to the pediatric population is *McCune-Albright syndrome*. This syndrome is rare and is suspected when a person has polyostotic fibrous dysplasia (malformation of bones), café-au-lait spots (light brown birthmarks), and endocrinopathies (various endocrine diseases). The most common endocrinopathy is precocious puberty, but hyperthyroidism also can be observed. In addition to other signs and symptoms of hyperthyroidism, patients initially present with a diffuse goiter that may become nodular over time. Unlike the hyperthyroidism of Graves' disease, McCune-Albright syndrome does not spontaneously go away and treatment with antithyroid medications provides only temporary benefit. Therefore, the treatment of choice is surgical resection or radioactive iodine ablation.

THYROID DISEASE AND PREGNANCY

The relationship of thyroid disease and pregnancy is important for several reasons. First, pregnancy alters thyroid physiology and increases overall circulating concentrations of thyroid hormones. Also, pregnancy is associated with general immunosuppression, which causes an amelioration of symptoms that are associated with autoimmune thyroid diseases. Unfortunately, after the pregnancy is over (post-partum), people with previously asymptomatic autoimmune-mediated thyroid disease may develop symptoms of hyperthyroidism or hypothyroidism. Finally, it is estimated the 2–15 percent of women become hyperthyroid in post-partum, but this is generally self-limiting and transiently lasts for only several months.

REFERENCES

Altman, L. K. (1991). *"Clue to Bushes' disease sought in water."* New York Times. NY.
Hull, G. (1998). "Caleb Hillier Parry 1755–1822: a notable provincial physician." *J R Soc Med* **91**(6): 335–8.

James, F., and R. J. J. Toole, Ed. (2001). Papers, Discussions, and Recommendations on the Twenty-Fifth Amendment and Issues of Inability and Disability in Presidents of the United States. Rochester, NY, University of Rochester Press,.

Sawin, C. T. (2002). "The heritage of Dr. Hakaru Hashimoto (1881–1934)." *Endocr J* **49**(4): 399–403.

Takami, H. E., and R. Miyabe, et al. (2008). "Hashimoto's thyroiditis." *World J Surg* **32**(5): 688–92.

4

Thyroid Nodules and Thyroid Goiter

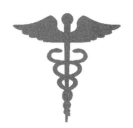

THYROID GOITER: A WORLDWIDE PROBLEM

So far we have learned about some of the conditions which affect the function of the thyroid. In some cases there can be actual enlargement of the thyroid. This enlargement of the thyroid is called a *goiter*. Thyroid goiters have been around a long time and were first described more than 3,000 years ago (see details on the historical importance of goiters in Chapter 1). Most goiters start out as painless symmetric enlargements of the thyroid but can progress with development of multiple lumps which are called *thyroid nodules*, this conditions is named *multinodular goiter*. In some cases these nodules may eventually start to be the cause of hyperthyroidism, this is called *toxic multinodular goiter* (discussed in detail in Chapter 3). Some simple indications may make people wonder if their thyroid is enlarged: it might be hard to button up a collar on a shirt or friends or family might notice that a person's neck looks thicker or wider than usual. Sometimes, doctors will comment on a goiter when they examine the neck during a routine physical examination. In many cases, the goiter will slowly grow and become quite prominent.

Worldwide iodine deficiency is the most common cause of simple goiter, but it can also occur in areas where there is an anti-thyroid or goiter-producing compounds (goiterogens) in the daily diet. Goiterogens are special chemicals found in certain foods that interfere with the body's ability to properly use iodine to synthesize thyroid hormone. Since iodine is essential for the thyroid to make thyroid hormone, a short supply of iodine causes increased TSH, stimulation and enlargement of the thyroid gland as it tries to compensate. As the thyroid enlarges, most of the time it is in fact able to maintain normal levels of thyroid hormone but at a cost: an enlarged thyroid which over time can become a nuisance. As the thyroid responds to the iodine deficiency with enlargement, parts of the thyroid become discrete nodules or lumps. Over the years, some of these nodules can become quite large so the entire thyroid consists of nodules of varying size. Worldwide over 750 million people suffer from iodine deficiency and thus goiters are very common the whole world over!

Iodine, a mineral found in seawater is essential for normal function of the thyroid. Humans don't make any iodine, so iodine needs to enter their body from the foods they eat. Normally when seawater evaporates and makes rain, the rain lands on soil where it is stored and ends up in certain foods, mostly milk, eggs, and certain vegetables. Iodine deficiency is common in areas far removed from the sea such as around the Great Lakes region of the United States, the Alps in Europe, the Himalayas in Asia, the Andes mountains in South America, as well as certain landlocked areas of Iran, China, Africa, and New Guinea. While a given human being only needs one teaspoon of iodine for their entire lifetime, even that can be hard to come by. Soil erosion, deforestation and overgrazing also contribute to low levels of iodine in the salt.

In areas with low iodine content in the food, goiter is *endemic*, meaning over 20 percent of the population suffers from it. The less iodine present in a given geographic location, the higher the number of people affected by goiter. Keep in mind that in some places over 90 percent of the population has goiters. Unfortunately once the process of thyroid enlargement starts, giving iodine will not reverse the process, in fact it might be harmful and dangerous. It is important to start out with an adequate level of iodine in the diet to prevent enlargement before it poses a major health risk. Given the importance of iodine to the general population's thyroid and the extra added importance in women who are pregnant or breastfeeding, many countries including the United States have supplemented salt sold in the country with iodine for over four to five decades. In fact, in the United States, additional iodine is also placed in animal feed, fertilizers, and preservatives. This interesting public health issue was discussed in detail in Chapter 2.

There are some rare cases where people have plenty of iodine in their diet, but due to some kind of problem with synthesis in their thyroid cells, they cannot make thyroid hormone. These conditions are quite unusual, often run in families, and

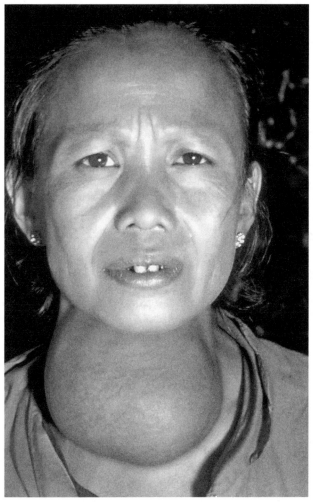

Large goiter seen in a woman. Endemic goiter continues to be a worldwide problem due to iodine deficiency. (Lester V. Bergman/Corbis)

usually present in childhood or even at birth when the baby is noted to have an enlarged thyroid. Giving thyroid hormone will usually significantly shrink the goiter in these unusual cases.

Most small goiters are barely noticed by the person and no treatment is needed; if the person is iodine deficient, iodized salt should be added to the diet and used in cooking. It is important not to take in too much iodine or eat certain iodine-containing foods such as kelp and seaweed, since too much iodine can further increase the size of the goiter. Sometimes if the goiter is small, low dose synthetic thyroid hormone is given to see if this will keep the goiter at a small size. This tends to work in some but not all people.

Most often, if the goiter enlarges, it usually will come to medical attention because it causes pressure symptoms in the neck or because nodules develop in the thyroid. Some people can get such massive thyroid enlargement that some parts of the thyroid crawl under the collar bone and end up in the chest next to the lungs; this is called a *substernal goiter*, since the thyroid is found under the chest bone (sternum). Very large goiters can even block blood flow draining out of the head and neck causes facial flushing when the arms are raised, this is called *Pemberton's Sign*, after Dr. Hugh Pemberton who first described it. The good news is that thyroid goiters rarely become cancerous, though they should all be watched for signs of certain characteristics which might signal *malignant degeneration*. Very large goiters sometimes need to be removed with surgery.

THYROID NODULES: BIG LUMPS, LITTLE LUMPS

Thyroid nodules are lumps found in the thyroid gland and are much more common than once thought. Nodules can range in size from several millimeters to many centimeters. Very large nodules may replace nearly half the thyroid and are visible to the naked eye. Very small thyroid nodules detected on a neck ultrasound are unlikely to be of any clinical significance. Physicians will perform further evaluation of small thyroid nodules if the patient has a family history of thyroid cancer, history of radiation exposure, or concomitant enlarged lymph nodes. When larger thyroid nodules are detected (generally greater than one centimeter), evaluation is usually warranted to rule out a cancer. The majority of thyroid nodules are benign (over 90%). Some patients have a thyroid goiter with multiple nodules throughout the thyroid (multinodular goiter); these nodules are almost always benign.

Thyroid nodules are a common condition seen worldwide: 10–40 percent of the population will develop a thyroid nodule during their lifetime (Gharib, Papini et al. 2008). Although common throughout all populations, thyroid nodules are most common in women. One third of women who receive a neck ultrasound have detectable thyroid nodules. While thyroid nodules are common, thyroid cancer is a rare disease, only approximately 15,000–20,000 cases are diagnosed each year in the United States. Evaluation of a thyroid nodule varies by physician preference but there are some general guidelines that need to be followed (Cooper, Doherty et al. 2009). When a thyroid nodule is detected, the physician will ask about the patient's medical history and perform a complete physical exam. Symptoms such as pain, swelling in the neck, difficulty with swallowing, shortness of breath, difficulty with breathing, or a change in the patient's voice should be discussed. Discussion of the patient's family history is important as some thyroid cancers are *familial*, which means it "runs in the family."

EVALUATING A THYROID NODULE: *THE IMPORTANT QUESTION—IS IT CANCER OR NOT?*

There are several steps that allow physicians to effectively evaluate and diagnose a patient's thyroid nodule. The first steps are taking a thorough history and examining the person. Things that make a doctor suspicious of that a nodule may harbor cancer.

Include:

Findings in the patient's history:
Rapid growth
Family history of a type of thyroid cancer called medullary carcinoma of the thyroid
Family history of a condition known as Multiple Endocrine Neoplasia 2 (MEN-2)
Young age (less than 20 yrs old)
Male gender
History of head or neck irradiation
Compressive symptoms such as problems swallowing or breathing

Findings upon examination of the patient:
Large nodule (greater than 4 cm in size)
A texture that is rock hard
Fixation of the nodule to surrounding structures such as neck muscles or the windpipe
Paralyzed vocal cord or hoarseness
A lot of difficulty with swallowing
Enlarged lymph nodes

Once the history and exam are over, tests may be ordered which can include:

Blood Tests

Blood tests measuring levels of thyroid hormone (free T4 and free T3) and thyroid stimulating hormone (TSH) may be performed. TSH is made by specialized cells in the pituitary gland, inside the brain (see Chapter 2 for details). If the level of thyroid hormone in the body drops, more TSH is made. This TSH in turn stimulates the thyroid gland to temporarily produce more hormone. This feedback loop makes TSH measurements very accurate in assessing the thyroid's function. In some cases, specialized testing of thyroid antibodies or thyroid stimulating immunoglobulins may be indicated. This is done if the physician suspects thyroiditis or autoimmune diseases of the thyroid (Graves' disease or Hashimoto's thyroiditis) as the cause for formation of the nodule. Currently no blood test exists for detecting the most common thyroid cancers. Thyroglobulin levels in the blood may be measured in patients with known cancers after removal of the thyroid to assess for any residual disease. Calcitonin is a blood test that is used to detect patients who may have medullary carcinoma of the thyroid (a rare kind of thyroid cancer). Calcitonin is a 32-amino acid linear polypeptide hormone produced primarily by the parafollicular cells (also known as C-cells) of the thyroid. In humans, its function is usually not very significant but it is thought to reduce blood calcium levels (Ca^{2+}), opposing the effects of parathyroid hormone (PTH). It used as a marker of medullary thyroid cancer when elevated in the blood.

Genetic Testing

In some familial cases of thyroid cancer, genetic testing is necessary. Most genetic testing for thyroid cancer is done for certain inherited mutations that cause susceptibility to medullary thyroid cancer. These sets of mutations can also lead to other tumors in endocrine glands such as the adrenal, pancreas, pituitary or parathyroids. While these syndromes are quite rare, it is imperative that those families with the mutations be found since early intervention often saves the lives of those treated at an earlier stage.

Ultrasound

A thyroid *ultrasound* is a non-invasive imaging study used to see the thyroid gland as well as any adjacent lymph nodes. Sound waves are used to see an accurate picture of the whole thyroid. Nodules in the thyroid can be seen, the *ultrasonographer* can tell if the nodule is solid or cystic and the size and exact location of all the nodules. Ultrasound is not capable of detecting cancerous from non-cancerous nodules. Many physicians will use ultrasound in combination with a procedure to sample the cells inside the nodule to help determine the diagnosis. Ultrasounds can be performed by a radiologist, endocrinologist, or surgeon (Solorzano, Carneiro et al. 2004) and can be done as an outpatient. It is not painful and there is no radiation and relative to many of the imaging tools it is fairly inexpensive. It

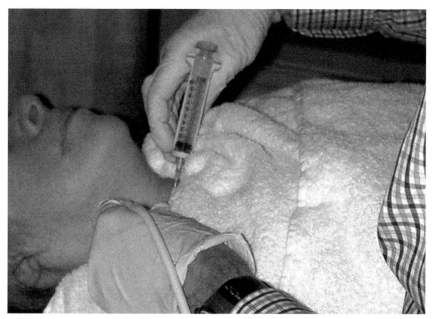

Fine needle aspiration of the thyroid under ultrasound guidance is often the first step in the work up of a thyroid nodule. (Courtesy of Dr. Sareh Parangi, MD)

appears to be the ideal tool for looking at what is going on inside the thyroid gland for the most part (Baskin 2004).

Fine Needle Aspiration (FNA)

Fine needle aspiration is removal of a small cluster of cells or fluid from the thyroid nodule using a very small needle attached to a syringe. Local anesthetic is sometimes used to numb or deaden the area of the biopsy though it is not always necessary. This procedure is safe and can be performed in the office of the physician. These cells are analyzed under a microscope by an experienced *cytologist* (a doctor specializing in pathology who has extra training to look at individual clusters of cells) and categorized as benign or malignant. It is not always possible to make a decision despite accurate or multiple fine needle aspirations.

The cytologist looks at the cells under the microscope similarly to PAP smears which are done routinely to screen for cervical cancer. When the cytologist looks at the fixed thyroid cells, they are specifically looking at several components of the biopsy including any background inflammatory changes, cellularity, architectural patterns, and cellular detail. Looking at thyroid cells is very difficult, and it is a mix of art and science, the pathologist then sends a report of the biopsy results to the physician who performed the biopsy. This report can detail four possible results.

Inadequate biopsy: this means not enough cells were withdrawn at the time of the biopsy and it is impossible for the cytologist to make any recommendations. In other words, the cytologist does not have enough information, they usually need at least six clusters of cells to tell is if a malignancy is present or not. The biopsy may be inadequate for many reasons including not having enough thyroid cells or presence of too much blood cells or cyst material to visualize the thyroid cells. A repeat biopsy is therefore indicated and may yield adequate material in at least 50 percent of repeat fine-needle aspiration biopsies. If the repeat biopsy is also inadequate, then the physician should discuss the benefits of trying a third biopsy versus referral to an endocrine surgeon for removal of the thyroid nodule.

Benign biopsy: this result means the cytologist saw multiple clusters of benign or non-cancerous cells in the sampling from the thyroid nodule. This is the most common results, over 90–95 percent of all thyroid biopsies performed in the United States come back with benign non worrisome thyroid cells. These cells encompass many thyroid conditions discussed in this book including subacute granulomatous thyroiditis, Hashimoto's thyroiditis, Riedel's thyroiditis, adenomatoid nodule, and cellular adenomatoid nodule. In general what this means is that the lump in the thyroid contains basically normal thyroid cells which may be inflamed or slightly overgrown but are not cancerous. It is important to realize that a benign biopsy result is not an absolute guarantee that the entire thyroid nodule is not cancerous. The larger the thyroid nodule, the greater the chance that there may be a false negative biopsy or sampling error. A false negative biopsy means that the biopsy missed the cancerous portion of the nodule. Large thyroid nodules should be followed closely with neck ultrasound and repeat biopsy if any worrisome characteristics develop.

Malignant biopsy (positive for malignancy): This result means based on the cells the cytologist saw under the microscopy, he or she thinks with near 100 percent certainty that the nodule in the thyroid is cancerous. Usually several features of thyroid cancer have to be present in the cells for this diagnosis to be confirmed. Often the cytologist can not only tell the doctor that the nodule is cancerous, but they can give many more details including the type of cancer. Common cancers that can be fairly easily diagnosed on needle biopsy include: papillary carcinoma, medullary carcinoma, anaplastic carcinoma, and thyroid lymphoma. Chapter 5 will examine each of these types of thyroid cancer in more detail.

Indeterminate biopsy (Follicular neoplasm or atypical biopsy): This "gray zone" means the cytologist cannot really tell if there is a thyroid cancer, but the cells are slightly suspicious or atypical; they are not normal. The nodule could be a benign tumor or a cancerous tumor. An inherent limitation of fine-needle aspiration biopsies is that they cannot distinguish follicular adenoma from follicular carcinoma or Hürthle cell adenoma from Hürthle cell carcinoma. The reason for this limitation is that the diagnosis of follicular or Hürthle cell carcinoma requires the presence of invasion of the thyroid capsule or nearby blood vessels. The diagnosis of capsular or vascular invasion requires the entire thyroid nodule be removed and compared to the surrounding normal thyroid tissue. Therefore surgical excision of the thyroid nodule will be necessary to exclude a diagnosis of thyroid cancer. In general, an indeterminate follicular neoplasm has a 20–25 percent chance of being a follicular carcinoma, and an indeterminate Hürthle cell neoplasm has a 10–15 percent chance of being an Hürthle cell carcinoma. Some indeterminate biopsies on the other hand can be quite suspicious to the cytologist and they usually call these "suspicious but not diagnostic for malignancy." This suspicious result usually alerts the physician that there are many but not all the signs of malignancy in the sampled cells. In this case, many times the chance of malignancy approaches 50–65 percent and a total thyroidectomy is sometimes recommended.

Thyroid Scan (Radionuclide Imaging)

A form of nuclear medicine imaging in which radiopharmaceuticals are taken internally, for example intravenously or orally. Then, external detectors (gamma cameras) capture and form images from the radiation emitted by the radiopharmaceuticals. This process is unlike a diagnostic X-ray where external radiation is passed through the body to form an image. Diagnostic tests in nuclear medicine exploit the way that the body handles substances differently when there is disease or pathology present. The radionuclide introduced into the body is often chemically bound to a complex that acts characteristically within the body; this is commonly known as a tracer. In the presence of disease, a tracer will often be distributed around the body and/or processed differently. These tests generally look at the function of the thyroid gland by measuring how much iodine it can take up from the bloodstream in a set period of time. A thyroid scan is performed to see if the nodule is functioning and producing too much thyroid hormone (a hot nodule) or non-functioning and hardly producing any (cold nodule). Most hot nodules are benign and generally cold nodules have a higher chance of being malignant (see Figure 4.1).

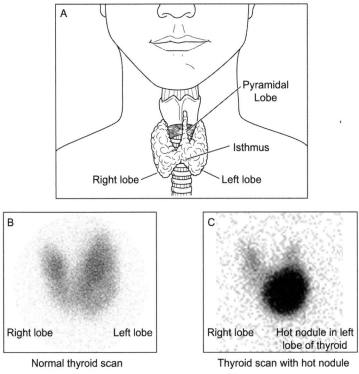

Figure 4.1   Thyroid radionuclide scanning in a patient with hyperthyroidism reveals one single "hot" nodule as the cause of the increased thyroid hormone production and hyperthyroidism. (Drawn by Jeff Dixon)

Magnetic Resonance Imaging (MRI) or Computed Tomography (CT Scan)

These specialized imaging techniques produce high quality pictures of the thyroid which are needed very rarely. For most thyroid nodules or even thyroid cancers, ultrasound imaging of the thyroid is far superior to these more expensive techniques (Haber 2000; Deandrea, Mormile et al. 2002). CAT scans use ionizing radiation to take precise thin cut pictures of the neck and thyroid gland which can then be put back together using computers. CAT scans are rarely used as a first tool in imaging the thyroid, since it is not very good at discerning differences between benign and cancerous growths in the thyroid. This test is very good at looking for enlarged thyroid goiters that have crept under the collarbone or in those with very large cancers which may be attached to other nearby organs. MRIs are a common but relatively new radiologic imaging modality used to visualize detailed internal structure and limited function of the body. A MRI provides much greater contrast and details between the different soft tissues of the body than computed axial tomography (CAT) does for some body parts especially the brain. A MRI uses no ionizing radiation but uses a powerful magnetic field to align hydrogen atoms in water in the body. Radiofrequency fields are used to systematically alter the alignment of this magnetization, causing the hydrogen nuclei to produce a rotating magnetic field detectable by the scanner. This signal can be manipulated by additional magnetic fields to build up enough information to construct an image of the body. MRIs are also rarely used for those with thyroid problems. Some surgeons use this tool to look for lymph nodes which might be hiding cancer cells.

TREATMENT OF THYROID NODULES: SIMPLE TO COMPLICATED

Depending on the specific thyroid nodule, treatment varies from simple monitoring to surgery. Much of the decision-making depends on the results of the ultrasound and any diagnostic tests such as the fine needle aspiration biopsy. Some of the decision making also depends on the comfort level of the patient with a particular strategy. In fact deciding what to do with a particular nodule is so complicated that many of the thyroid specialists (see list in Chapter 2) came together for an entire year to work together to issue comprehensive guidelines on the work up of thyroid nodules (Cooper, Doherty et al. 2009). In cases of noncancerous or multiple nodules, thyroid hormone replacement may stop further growth or shrink the nodules. If patients choose not to take hormones, they may opt for serial follow up ultrasounds (usually once every six months to a year) and additional periodic biopsies. The frequency of follow up will depend on factors including the patient's medical and family history, how big the nodule is, how quickly it grew, and results of the physician evaluations.

If the results of testing lead to suspicion of a tumor or cancer of the thyroid, surgery to remove part or the entire thyroid may be recommended. In some cases thyroid surgery is best done sooner rather than waiting until the nodule becomes larger. All of these options are discussed in detail in Chapters 5 and 6.

REFERENCES

Baskin, H. J. (2004). "Thyroid ultrasound-just do it." *Thyroid* **14**(2): 91–2.

Cooper, D. S., G. M. Doherty, et al. (2009). "Revised American Thyroid Association management guidelines for patients with thyroid nodules and differentiated thyroid cancer." *Thyroid* **19**(11): 1167–214.

Deandrea, M., A. Mormile, et al. (2002). "Fine-needle aspiration biopsy of the thyroid: comparison between thyroid palpation and ultrasonography." *Endocr Pract* **8**(4): 282–86.

Gharib, H., E. Papini, et al. (2008). "Thyroid nodules: a review of current guidelines, practices, and prospects." *Eur J Endocrinol* **159**(5): 493–505.

Haber, R. S. (2000). "Role of ultrasonography in the diagnosis and management of thyroid cancer." *Endocr Pract* **6**(5): 396–400.

Solorzano, C. C., D. M. Carneiro, et al. (2004). "Surgeon-performed ultrasound in the management of thyroid malignancy." *Am Surg* **70**(7): 576–80; discussion 580–2.

5

Thyroid Cancer

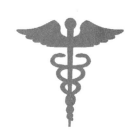

THYROID CANCER: THE "C" WORD

Most people are scared of the "C" word, and having cancer or knowing of a family member with cancer can be a scary experience. Cancer is a complex collection of diseases that feature unregulated or uncontrolled cellular growth. Normal body cells have a well-regulated system of cellular growth, cellular division, and then eventually cellular death. Adult cells typically reproduce only to replace worn-out or injured cells. On the other hand, cancer cells become "immortal" in the sense that they ignore normal cellular growth controls and continue to grow and divide even at the expense of surrounding cells. Non-blood cancer cells cluster together and eventually form a detectable lump once there are at least a billion cancer cells. Cancer cells may also acquire the ability to travel to other parts of the body and forming new colonies of cancer cells. This process of moving to other parts of the body is called *metastasis*, which is a derivation of the Greek word "methistanai," which means, "to change."

The National Cancer Institute keeps track of various statistics related to many different cancers, and some important ones regarding all kinds of thyroid cancers are listed here. Thyroid cancer is less common than many other types of cancer and represents only one percent of all new cancers diagnosed in the United States each year (approximately 24,000 people) (see Graph 5.1).

Annual Incidence of Cancers
(Cases per 100,000)

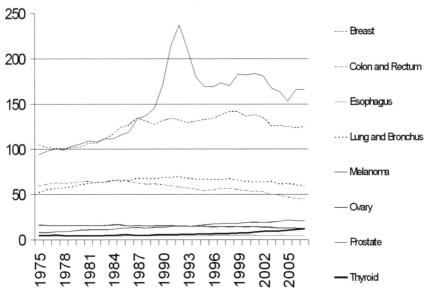

Graph 5.1   Incidence of thyroid cancer relative to other cancers in the United States. (*Source*: Altekruse SF 2010)

- *Incidence* of a cancer means the risk of developing some new condition within a specified period of time. The overall incidence of thyroid cancer is ~10/100,000 per year which means that ten people in every 100,000 people in the United States will be diagnosed with thyroid cancer each year. The incidence of thyroid cancer also increases with a person's age, which likely is a reflection of the time that it takes for new cancers to grow to a size that is detectable on clinical examination. In general, thyroid cancer is significantly less common than some other cancers, but in women it is a pretty common cancer. According to the most recent data in the Surveillance and Epidemiology End Results (SEER) database from the National Institute of Health, the age-adjusted incidence rate of thyroid cancer was 10.2 per 100,000 men and women per year. These rates are based on cases diagnosed in 2000–2007 from 17 SEER geographic areas (see Graph 5.2).

  From 2003 to 2007, the median age at diagnosis for cancer of the thyroid was 49 years of age. Approximately 1.8 percent of all thyroid cancers were diagnosed under age 20; 16.3 percent between 20 and 34; 21.5 percent between 35 and 44; 24.1 percent between 45 and 54; 17.6 percent between

Age-Specific Incidence Rates
(Cases per 100,000, 2000-2007)

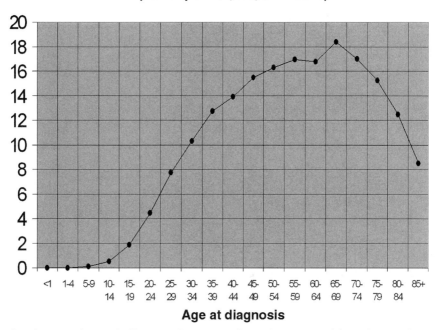

Age at diagnosis

Graph 5.2   This graph illustrates the age-specific incidence rates of thyroid cancer from 2000 to 2007. Note how thyroid cancer is most common in people who are between 60 and 70 years old.

55 and 64; 11.2 percent between 65 and 74; 6.1 percent between 75 and 84; and 1.4 percent 85+ years of age (Altekruse SF 2010). However, the incidence of thyroid cancer has been steadily rising over the last several decades for reasons that are not completely clear (see Graph 5.3). One frequently cited reason is the increase in imaging of the thyroid gland and therefore the detection of small papillary thyroid cancers (Davies and Welch 2006).

However, two recent studies have noted an increase in all size thyroid cancers, which suggests that environmental, dietary, or genetic factors may be involved (Chen, Jemal et al. 2009; Enewold, Zhu et al. 2009). These factors may include the rising body mass index, insulin-resistance syndrome, and the use of fertility medications (Goodman, Kolonel et al. 1992; Engeland, Tretli et al. 2006; Hannibal, Jensen et al. 2008; Rezzonico, Rezzonico et al. 2008). Thyroid cancer occurs in women three times more frequently compared to men and is most commonly diagnosed in the third to fourth decades of life.

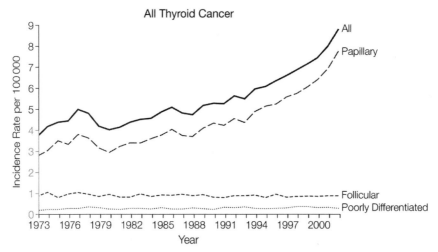

Graph 5.3   Incidence of thyroid cancer from 1973 to 2006.
(*Source:* Reproduced with permission from Davies L, Welch HG. "Increasing incidence of thyroid cancer in the United States, 1973–2002." *JAMA*, 2006 May 10; 295(18):2164–67. Copyright ©(2006) American Medical Association. All rights reserved.)

- *Survival* can be calculated by different methods for different purposes. Calculating survival rates means using biostatistics to figure out the percentage of people in a study or treatment group who are alive for a given period of time after diagnosis. Whether a type of cancer has a good or bad prognosis can be determined from its survival rate. Prognosis is often expressed over standard time periods, like one, five, and ten years. For example thyroid cancer has a much better prognosis than pancreatic cancer because the five-year survival from thyroid cancer is basically close to 95 percent whereas the five-year survival for pancreatic cancer is closer to 5–10 percent. When someone is more interested in how survival is affected by the disease, there is also the net survival rate, which filters out the effect of mortality from other causes than the disease. The two main ways to calculate net survival are *relative survival* and *disease specific survival.* Relative survival is calculated by dividing the overall survival after diagnosis of a disease by the survival as observed in a similar population that was not diagnosed with that disease. A similar population is composed of individuals with at least age and gender similar to those diagnosed with the disease. Disease specific survival is calculated by treating deaths from causes other than the disease as withdrawals from the population that don't lower survival, comparable to patients who are not observed any longer, e.g., due to reaching the end of the study period. Relative survival has the advantage that it does not depend on accuracy of

Five-Year Survival Rate by Race and Sex (Percent)

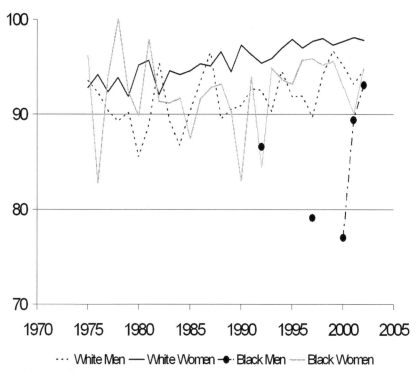

··· White Men — White Women –•· Black Men –– Black Women

Graph 5.4   This graph illustrates the overall 5-year relative thyroid cancer survival by race and gender based on the year of diagnosis. Note that overall survival has improved in all groups of patients since the 1970s.

the reported cause of death; disease specific survival has the advantage that it does not depend on the ability to find a similar population of people without the disease.

The survival statistics presented here for thyroid cancer are based on relative survival, which measures the survival of the cancer patients in comparison to the general population to estimate the effect of cancer. The overall five-year relative survival for 1999–2006 from 17 SEER geographic areas was 97.3 percent. Five-year relative survival by race and sex from 1975 to 2002 was: 94.6 percent for white men; 98.2 percent for white women; 90.9 percent for black men; 95.4 percent for black women (see Graph 5.4) (Altekruse SF 2010).

- *Prevalence* is an epidemiologic term which is defined as the total number of cases of the disease in the population at a given time, or the total number of cases in the population, divided by the number of individuals in the population. It is used as an estimate of how common a condition is within a population over a certain period of time. It helps doctors or other health professionals understand the probability of certain diseases such as cancer, including thyroid cancer. The most recent available SEER data on the prevalence of thyroid cancer shows that on January 1, 2007, in the United States there were approximately 434,256 people alive who had a history of cancer of the thyroid—96,230 men and 338,026 women. This includes any person alive on January 1, 2007, who had been diagnosed with cancer of the thyroid at any point prior to January 1, 2007, and includes persons with active disease and those who are cured of their disease.

Thyroid cancers can arise from any of the cells that are present in the normal thyroid gland. Most thyroid cancers are derived from the most common kind of cells in the thyroid: the follicular cells. Cancers derived from the thyroid follicular cells are either *well-differentiated* or *undifferentiated* carcinomas. The two types of well-differentiated thyroid cancers are papillary and follicular carcinomas and the only type of undifferentiated carcinoma is anaplastic carcinoma.

Cancers from the calcitonin-producing C *cell* in the thyroid is called medullary thyroid carcinoma (MTC). The relative frequency of each type of thyroid cancer is illustrated in Graph 5.3, but as a general rule of thumb: most thyroid cancers are papillary thyroid cancer (luckily also happens to be the one with the best outcome) and the next most common is follicular thyroid cancer. Medullary thyroid cancer, anaplastic thyroid cancer, and thyroid lymphoma are much rarer, which is a good thing because they are generally harder to treat and patients tend to not do quite as well.

THE NATURAL HISTORY OF THYROID CANCER: FROM NORMAL TO CANCEROUS, IT DOESN'T HAPPEN OVERNIGHT!

Thyroid cancers likely start as normal thyroid cells that are somehow influenced to transform into malignant cancer cells. Influences on a normal cell that can cause a transformation from normal to cancerous include: genetic, environmental, nutritional, chemical, radiation, or traumatic. Thyroid cells are no different. Some people are genetically predisposed to thyroid cancer because they inherited some genes that eventually lead to thyroid cancer; others start with genetically normal cells but over their lifetime the cells accumulate genetic "hits" or damage due to certain environmental, nutritional, or chemical influences. One very important and well studied example cause of damage to thyroid cells is radiation, and this well be discussed in detail later in this chapter. Surely there are numerous other reasons thyroid cells "go bad," many of which have not been discovered or studied yet, leaving ample room for future studies.

HOW THYROID CANCERS ARE FOUND: THE SILENT EPIDEMIC

Thyroid cancers are often found one of two ways. Many thyroid cancers are detected when a person or health-care provider feels a painless nodule in the central portion of the neck. Remember that nodule is a fancy word for a lump in the thyroid. If an experienced health professional examined everyone in the United States, they would find palpable thyroid nodules in about 20 percent of the population (Ezzat, Sarti et al. 1994). However, only a small number of those thyroid nodules (probably <10%) would have a cancer inside of them. Certain elements in a patient's history or story about the thyroid nodule can make a physician more worried that the thyroid nodule may have cancer. These elements include male gender, a history of head or neck irradiation, age less than 20 or over 45 years, family history of thyroid cancer, a hoarse voice, large nodule size (>4 cm), the nodule seems to be attached to nearby structures in the neck, and the thyroid nodule is getting larger over a short period of time (Hegedus 2004). Having some or all of these things makes a health-care provider more suspicious of thyroid cancer.

DIAGNOSING THYROID CANCER: FINDING THE NEEDLE IN THE HAYSTACK

Finding the thyroid cancer among all the thyroid nodules out there, the numbers can be staggering. Lots of people have thyroid nodules (millions), often one person can even have multiple thyroid nodules. The good news is that most thyroid nodules are benign with only about 5–10 percent of all nodules containing a cancer. What is a doctor to do? Doctors have to try and use information about each patient and each nodule to help ascertain whether a particular nodule is cancerous. Physicians may perform studies to help determine which nodules contain cancer. The most common and by far the two most informative tests are an ultrasound of the thyroid and a fine-needle aspiration biopsy test with or without ultrasound guidance. The ultrasound visualizes the entire thyroid and any nodules in it. While most doctors cannot tell whether a particular nodule is cancerous based on ultrasound alone, certain ultrasound features of thyroid nodules make it more suspicious. For example, if the nodule appears "*hypoechoic*" or darker than normal surrounding thyroid tissue, has small calcium deposits called *calcifications*, or has lots of blood flowing into the lump from every direction. Thyroid nodules that are larger than 1.5–2 cm, have suspicious features on ultrasound, or are present in a patient with major physical signs of thyroid cancer such as hoarseness or enlarged lymph nodes, need to be biopsied to allow a sampling of the cells that are found inside the lump. This test can be done in a physician's office and involves placing a very small needle into the thyroid nodule using a local anesthetic to obtain a small sample of cells from that nodule. These cells are sent to a pathologist or cytologist in a special preservative solution and examined under a microscope to determine if the biopsy contains cancerous cells. This is very similar to the techniques used in a PAP smear which are done routinely to screen for cervical cancer. When the pathologist looks at the fixed thyroid cells, they are specifically looking at several components of the biopsy including any background inflammatory changes, cellularity, architectural patterns, and cellular detail. Looking at thyroid cells under the microscope to differentiate between benign and cancerous conditions is very difficult. The pathologist then sends a report of the biopsy results to the physician who performed the biopsy. This report can detail four possible results results.

The first result is that the biopsy is inadequate to determine if malignancy is present or not. The biopsy may be inadequate for many reasons including not having enough thyroid cells or presence of too much blood cells or cyst material to visualize the thyroid cells. A repeat biopsy is therefore indicated and may yield adequate material in at least 50 percent of repeat fine-needle aspiration biopsies (Richards, Bohnenblust et al. 2008). If the repeat biopsy is also inadequate then the physician should discuss the benefits of trying a third biopsy versus referral to an endocrine surgeon for removal of the thyroid nodule.

The second possible biopsy result is that the thyroid nodule contains benign or non-cancerous cells. This is the most common result, over 90–95 percent of all thyroid biopsies performed in the United States come back with benign non worrisome thyroid cells. These cells encompass many thyroid conditions discussed in this book including subacute granulomatous thyroiditis, Hashimoto's thyroiditis, Riedel's thyroiditis, adenomatoid nodule, and cellular adenomatoid nodule. In general, this means that the lump in the thyroid basically contains normal thyroid cells, which may be inflamed or slightly overgrown but are not cancerous. It is important to realize that a benign biopsy result is not an absolute guarantee that the entire thyroid nodule is not cancerous. The larger the thyroid nodule, the greater the chance that there may be a false negative biopsy or sampling error which means that the biopsy missed the cancerous portion of the nodule. Large thyroid nodules should be followed closely with neck ultrasound and repeat biopsy if any worrisome characteristics develop.

The third possible biopsy result is called a malignant neoplasm. This means the pathologist thinks with near 100 percent certainty that the nodule in the thyroid is cancerous. Usually several features of thyroid cancer have to be present in the cells for this diagnosis to be confirmed. Often the pathologist can not only tell the doctor that the nodule is cancerous, but they can give many more details including the type of cancer. Common cancers that can be fairly easily diagnosed on needle biopsy include: papillary carcinoma, medullary carcinoma, anaplastic carcinoma, and thyroid lymphoma. The rest of this chapter will examine each type of thyroid cancer in more detail.

The fourth possible biopsy result is an indeterminate *neoplasm*. This "gray zone" means the pathologist cannot really tell if there is a thyroid cancer, but the cells are slightly suspicious or atypical; they are not normal. The nodule could be a benign tumor or a cancerous tumor. An inherent limitation of fine-needle aspiration biopsies is that they cannot distinguish follicular adenoma from follicular carcinoma or Hürthle cell adenoma from Hürthle cell carcinoma. The reason for this limitation is that the diagnosis of follicular or Hürthle cell carcinoma requires the presence of invasion of the thyroid capsule or nearby blood vessels. The diagnosis of capsular or vascular invasion requires the entire thyroid nodule be removed and compared to the surrounding normal thyroid tissue. Therefore surgical excision of the thyroid nodule will be necessary to exclude a diagnosis of thyroid cancer. In general, an indeterminate follicular neoplasm has a 20–25 percent chance of being a follicular carcinoma, and an indeterminate Hürthle cell neoplasm has a 10–15 percent chance of being an Hürthle cell carcinoma (Schlinkert, van Heerden et al. 1997).

WELL-DIFFERENTIATED THYROID CARCINOMA: THE BEST OF THE CANCERS

As mentioned previously, there are two types of well-differentiated thyroid cancers, papillary and follicular.

PAPILLARY THYROID CANCER: THE BEST OF THE BEST

Papillary thyroid cancer represents the vast majority of thyroid cancers (80% of all thyroid neoplasms) and may be *multicentric* (occur in multiple locations or in both thyroid lobes simultaneously). The development of papillary thyroid cancer is associated with radiation exposure and autoimmune thyroiditis (Hashimoto's thyroiditis), and typically spreads through the lymphatic networks of the body as opposed to the bloodstream or direct invasion. The lymph nodes that are most frequently involved are in the central compartment of the neck, which is the region of

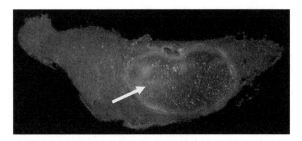

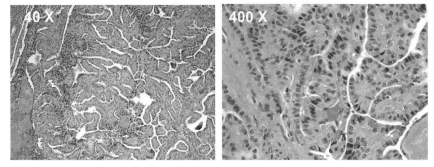

Papillary thyroid cancer in the thyroid lobe marked by a white arrow (top panel); the capsule of the cancer is visible as a white rim around the tumor. The lower panel shows papillary thyroid cancer magnified under the microscope 40 and 400 times. The nuclei of the thyroid cancer cells are quite different when compared to those in normal thyroid cells. (Courtesy of Peter Sadow and Dr. Sareh Parangi, MD)

the neck below the voice box, above the collarbones, and in between both carotid arteries. However, papillary thyroid cancer may spread to the lymph nodes on both sides of the neck as well, which are termed the lateral compartments. The good news is that papillary thyroid cancers are slow-growing so it is typically diagnosed before it has spread to other organs in the body (metastasis). Only 5–10 percent of people with papillary thyroid cancers develop distant metastases with the most common sites being either the lungs or bones (DeGroot, Kaplan et al. 1990).

RADIATION AND PAPILLARY THYROID CANCER: TISK, TISK, TISK . . . WHAT YOU CAN'T SEE CAN HURT YOU

The greatest risk factor for the development of papillary thyroid cancer is head or neck radiation exposure, especially during childhood (Schneider and Sarne 2005). This was unfortunately a hard-learned lesson of the early twentieth century; the consequences of which we are still facing today. The story of how radiation exposure was linked to later development of thyroid cancer is a fascinating one indeed. Remember that radiation is energy that moves from one spot to another:

sunshine, heat, microwaves, gamma rays, and X-rays are all examples of radiation. Radiation energy waves are present all around us. Some types of radiation are weak and harmless, whereas others are quite powerful. *Ionizing radiation* occurs when an atom is given so much energy that electrons jump out of their normal orbit around the atom and then "crash" into human chromosomal structures. This damage leads to chromosomal breaks, which can lead to genetic rearrangements that stimulate uncontrolled cellular growth or permanently damage genes that prevent abnormal cellular growth called tumor-suppressor genes. So how would a person receive ionizing radiation? Although some people have occupational exposure to ionizing radiation (frequent high altitude flights, X-ray technician, etc.), other people may have been exposed before the true dangers of radiation were fully discovered (Boice and Lubin 1997). For example, in the 1920–1950s, children routinely

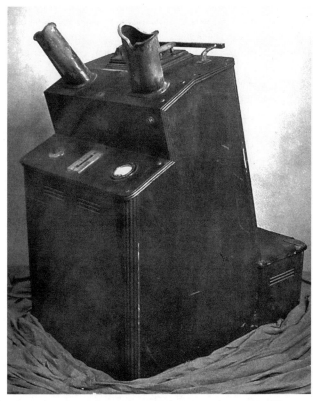

A standard Adrian shoe-fitting fluoroscope machine circa late 1930s. This type of machine would use X-rays to observe a child's foot moving inside of a shoe to ensure that the shoe had a "perfect fit." Unfortunately, these machines degraded over time and exposed customers and shoe salesmen to dangerous X-ray radiation. (National Library of Medicine)

One More Thing to Know: Now That's Interesting
How the Search for the Perfect Shoe Led to Thyroid Cancer

Can you imagine using X-rays to size your shoes? It seems like overkill now but in the 1920 amid the Great depression a special X-ray machine was used to size shoes exactly to individual feet, money was tight and it was thought to be an excellent way to save money by ensuring shoes had enough room for children to grow into. The shoe-fitting fluoroscope was a common instrument used in shoe stores around the world starting in the United States in the early 1920s. Although the exact origins of the shoe-fitting fluoroscope is not entirely clear, it was likely in part invented by a Boston physician named Dr. Jacob Lowe for use in World War I. Dr. Lowe used the device to examine soldier's feet for shrapnel or bony injuries without removing the soldier's boots. After the war, Dr. Lowe modified the device for shoe fitting and sold the patent to the Adrian Manufacturing Company.

A typical Adrian shoe-fitting machine is pictured in this chapter. It basically consisted of a wooden cabinet that had an X-ray tube at the base and a fluoroscopic screen at the top. The customer would place his/her feet into an opening at the bottom of the machine and then look through a viewport that connected to the fluoroscopic screen at the top of the machine. When the machine was activated, X-ray radiation would pass through the customer's feet and show the bones of the customer's foot and the outline of the shoe. Shoe-fitting fluoroscope companies claimed that seeing how the bones fit against the shoe would ensure a "perfect fit." This sales pitch proved popular and over 10,000 were sold in the United States alone, each for approximately $2,000.

Unfortunately, many of the now obvious dangers of radiation were still not understood when shoe fluoroscopes were popular. All of the new machines had a lead lining that prevented radiation from leaking out of the machine and onto the customer's face and neck. However, since many shoe store managers were not trained in servicing the shoe fluoroscopes, this lead lining eventually weakened and allowed radiation to bathe customers' thyroid glands.

After World War II, many medical professional organizations urged the state and federal governments to restrict the use of shoe fluoroscopes by non-medical personnel. In the late 1950s, the state of Pennsylvania became the first to outright ban the use of shoe-fitting fluoroscopes. Shoe-fitting fluoroscopes were phased out of shoe stores in the United States by the late 1960s, but were used in Canada and the United Kingdom until the 1970s. Ironically, despite exposing millions of customers and salespeople to unnecessary amounts of radiation, the shoe-fitting fluoroscope was never proven to result in a better fitting shoe than standard non-radioactive foot measurements.

received sizable doses of radiation from shoe-fitting fluoroscopes; this became a major risk factor for development of thyroid cancer in these children, sometimes 40–50 years later. Also, in the early 1950–1960s, it was not uncommon to receive head and neck irradiation as treatment for acne and tonsillitis.

Finally, during the Cold War between the United States and the former Soviet Union, workers in the nuclear industry occasionally received excessive amounts of occupational radiation exposure. Obviously, people who lived near nuclear reactor accident sites such as Chernobyl in the former Soviet Union, or Three-Mile Island in New York State are also at risk for developing papillary thyroid cancer (Boice and Lubin 1997).

What History Can Teach Us:
The Chernobyl Nuclear Disaster and Thyroid Cancer

In this era of nuclear bombs and nuclear energy, one of the most feared calamities is a nuclear accident. On the morning of April 28, 1986, the world woke up to the frightening news from behind the Iron Curtain of the Soviet Union: Two days prior and some 80 miles north of Kiev, the capital of Ukraine, the world's worst nuclear disaster had occurred in Unit 4 of the Chernobyl Nuclear Power Plant. The story of how this nuclear accident happened and its effects on the thyroid glands of hundreds of thousands of people is a good lesson to remember for everyone.

Ironically, the cause of this disaster was an experiment to try and prevent a catastrophic nuclear reactor meltdown. The day before the accident, Chernobyl engineers were eager to try an experiment to see if they could draw energy from the steam turbines, instead of diesel generators, to run water pumps in case of a nuclear emergency. To create the appropriate conditions for the experiment, many of the reactor's safety features were deactivated. Unfortunately, at 01:23 during the initial phase of the experiment, an uncontrolled nuclear chain reaction led to an enormous steam and chemical explosion that destroyed the reactor's closure head. The resulting damage exposed the superheated nuclear power core to the outside air. The power core immediately caused the air around the power plant to ignite into an enormous fire that ultimately burned for ten days. The combination of the initial explosion and subsequent fire, allowed various types of radioactive particles and vapors to enter the atmospheric air currents and spread over much of Europe.

Despite the enormous health risks, the government of the Soviet Union decided to contain any news of the Chernobyl disaster from Western media sources. News of Chernobyl was finally announced two days after the reactor explosions when Sweden found high levels of radiation emanating from the Ukraine. It is estimated that as much as 20 percent of these radioactive particles and vapors may have spread beyond Europe.

Ultimately, the five million people living within the "red zone" which included areas of Russia, Belarus, and the Ukraine, received the highest dosages of radioactivity. In addition, approximately 600,000 emergency and recovery operation workers were directly exposed during the subsequent containment efforts. The total cost of the accident over the last three decades has been estimated to be hundreds of billions of dollars and about 338,000 people had to be permanently relocated. The total release of radioactive substances was about 14 EBq, including 1.8 EBq of I^{131}, 0.085 EBq of Cs^{137}, 0.01 EBq of Sr^{90}, and 0.003 EBq of plutonium radioisotopes (Agency 2006).

The early months after the accident were characterized by surface deposition of I^{131} on agricultural plants and therefore inside plant-consuming animals. In particular, I^{131} was rapidly absorbed into cow's milk leading to very high dosages to people consuming milk, especially children (De Cort M 1998). Although the half-life of I^{131} is around eight days, a child's thyroid is particularly sensitive to radiation damage. Aggressive screening measures were started in all of the population areas affected by the Chernobyl radioactive fallout. From 1992 to 2002, approximately 4,000 cases of thyroid cancer have been diagnosed in individuals who were children at the time of the accident (Jacob, Bogdanova et al. 2006). Almost all of these cases have been papillary thyroid cancers. Since papillary thyroid cancers are very slow growing, it is likely that even more thyroid cancers caused by Chernobyl will be diagnosed over the next several decades.

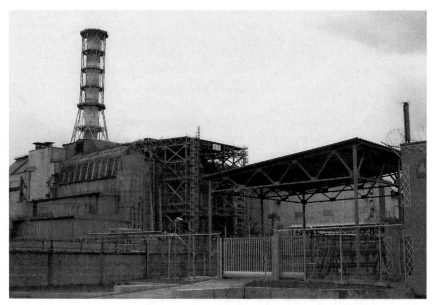

The Chernobyl nuclear power plant is located approximately 11 miles northwest of the city of Chernobyl near the border between the Ukraine and Belarus. On April 26, 1986, it was the site of a nuclear disaster that exposed millions of people to high levels of radioactive elements. (Shutterstock)

FOLLICULAR THYROID CANCER: JUST A LITTLE WORSE...

Follicular carcinoma is the other type of well-differentiated thyroid cancer and is a distant second-most common thyroid cancer representing ten percent of all thyroid cancers. People with follicular carcinoma are slightly older than people with papillary thyroid cancer, with the mean age at diagnosis in between the fourth and sixth decades of life. Follicular carcinoma is more common in regions of the world with iodine-deficiency for reasons that have not been completely elucidated. Unlike papillary thyroid cancer, follicular carcinoma rarely spreads to the lymph nodes, but can present with direct invasion into anatomical structures adjacent to the thyroid gland. If a follicular carcinoma invades into a person's trachea (windpipe), it can cause irritation leading the person to have hemoptysis (coughing spells with small amounts of bleeding). If the cancer invaded into the recurrent laryngeal nerve, a person may develop vocal cord paralysis on that side causing the person to have a hoarse, breathy-type voice and even dysphagia (difficulty swallowing food and/or liquids). Also, follicular carcinoma may spread to distant organs via the bloodstream at a significantly higher rate than papillary thyroid cancer (20% of all people with follicular carcinoma) (Grebe and Hay 1995).

Hürthle-cell thyroid carcinoma is a rare thyroid cancer that is currently considered a variant of follicular thyroid carcinoma. It is unique from other follicular thyroid carcinomas in that 75–100 percent of the tumor is composed of Hürthle cells. These cells are rotund, polygonal follicular cells that contain abundant cytoplasm, and can be found in a variety of benign thyroid conditions, such as Hashimoto thyroiditis, Graves' disease, and multinodular goiter. Hürthle-cell carcinomas account for two to three percent of all thyroid malignancies and are diagnosed most often in the fifth decade of life. Unlike papillary and follicular thyroid carcinomas, Hürthle-cell carcinomas are much more aggressive and are more likely to metastasize to distant organs (McHenry and Sandoval 1998).

TREATMENT OF WELL-DIFFERENTIATED THYROID CANCERS: THE FIRST STEP IS SURGERY

Once a well-differentiated thyroid cancer is diagnosed by fine-needle aspiration biopsy, the first and most important part of the treatment is almost always surgical removal of the thyroid. The surgeon has to decide on the kind of surgery that would most likely make sure the cancer is cured and does not recur. This usually means removal of the thyroid and possibly some lymph nodes in the vicinity of the thyroid.

As explained in detail later in Chapter 6, there are several different types of thyroid operations. The type of procedure surgeons choose depends on a number of factors: the patient's age and gender, size of the cancer in the thyroid, location of the cancer, details on the results of the fine needle aspiration, existence of enlarged lymph nodes in the neck, or a history of radiation. Surgeons decide with input from the patient and their endocrinologist which procedure is best suited to each patient's problem. Three kinds of thyroid surgery are commonly used and are listed here:

Thyroid lobectomy: One half of the thyroid is removed
Total thyroidectomy: The entire thyroid gland is removed
Lymph node dissection: Removal of some of some lymph nodes around the thyroid gland

Well-differentiated thyroid cancers are typically treated with removal of the entire thyroid gland, which is called a total thyroidectomy. Occasionally if the tumor is very small, removal of the half the thyroid gland, containing the cancerous nodule may be suggested, this is called a thyroid lobectomy or partial thyroidectomy. In the United States, most patients with thyroid cancer have the entire thyroid removed. Each treatment has its own benefits and risks. In experienced hands, total thyroidectomy is associated with a less than one percent chance of recurrent laryngeal nerve damage and a less than ten percent risk of permanent hypoparathyroidism (Hundahl, Cady et al. 2000). Permanent hypoparathyroidism usually results from injury to the parathyroid's blood supply during the operation and will require life-long vitamin D and calcium supplementation. Thyroid lobectomy has a lower incidence of recurrent laryngeal nerve damage or hypoparathyroidism compared to total thyroidectomy. However, removing only a portion of the thyroid means that a part of the cancer may still remain in the other thyroid lobe. It is also not possible to use radioactive iodine or thyroglobulin measurements post-operatively if only a portion of the thyroid is removed.

As discussed previously, thyroid cancer may spread to the surrounding lymph nodes in the lateral or central portion of the neck. If any abnormal lymph nodes are found on pre-operative ultrasound or during the operation, it may be necessary to also do a *lymphadenectomy* or excision of lymph nodes surrounding the thyroid. Some endocrine surgeons currently advocate lymphadenectomy of the central neck compartment in all patients with papillary thyroid cancer to decrease the chance that microscopic cancers may be present in an otherwise normal-appearing lymph node. Although this practice may decrease the incidence of subsequent lymph node metastases in the central neck, it does not appear to change the patient's overall disease course (Mazzaferri, Doherty et al. 2009).

TREATMENT OF WELL-DIFFERENTIATED THYROID CANCERS: HOW TO PREVENT RECURRENCES AFTER SURGERY

Radioiodine Treatment: The Search for the Magic Bullet?

Patients always want to know if their cancers could come back. This is a source of constant anxiety and worry, and thyroid cancer patients are no different. Doctors have developed some additional therapies against thyroid cancer cells which are actually quite innovative and unique. These therapies target thyroid cancer cells specifically using the natural affinity of all thyroid cells for iodine. As you recall from Chapter 2, iodine is an essential element for synthesis of thyroid hormone and each thyroid cell has a marked affinity for absorbing large amounts of thyroid hormone using specialized cellular pumps called *sodium-iodine symporters (NIS)*. Since well-differentiated thyroid cancers arise from the thyroid hormone-producing and thyroglobulin-producing follicular cells of the thyroid (see Chapter 2), thyroid cancer cells usually also have these specialized iodine receptors. Small amounts of radioactivity can be chemically bonded to iodine molecules to create iodine-131 (I-131) and then given to patients so that the radioactive iodine can be pulled into any normal or abnormal thyroid cells that might still be hiding in the body after thyroid surgery. Large doses of radioactivity can also be coupled to iodine molecules and once these special radioactive iodine molecules get into thyroid cells, they can kill that cell.

When physicians choose to give radioactive iodine, the patient often needs to stop their thyroid hormone and go on a low iodine diet. The purpose of stopping the thyroid hormone for 2–6 weeks prior to getting radioiodine treatment is to have a high Thyroid Stimulating Hormone (TSH) level. Remember that when thyroid hormone levels are very low, which happens when patients stop their thyroid hormone replacements after the thyroid has been surgically removed, the brain gets to work immediately secreting lots of TSH. This increase in TSH happens because of the special feedback loop in the hypothalamic-pituitary axis (see Chapter 2). When TSH is high, any remaining normal or abnormal thyroid cells in the body get "stimulated" and activate all their sodium-iodine symporters (NIS). This activation of all available NIS iodide pumps allows the maximum amount of radioactive iodine to be pumped into each thyroid cells thus making the treatment more likely to work in completely getting rid of all remaining normal or cancerous thyroid cells. The low iodine diet serves the same purpose, getting every pump hungry for iodine and ready to pump in the next batch of iodine that comes around (remember that the doctor is going to trick the cell by making it a radioactive batch of iodine instead of regular old iodine).

There are two basic ways to drive up the TSH in a patient with thyroid cancer. The high TSH is meant to promote uptake of the radioactive iodine into the thyroid cells. The traditional true and tested method, and the method still most often used the world over, is to withdraw the person from thyroid hormone for a few weeks (generally 2–6 weeks) and then do a blood test to see if the TSH in fact is very high. This works very well and often the TSH will go up to 60–80 μu/ml. Remember a normal TSH is somewhere under 4 μu/ml or so. The problem with this approach is that during the time the patient is off thyroid hormone, they usually experience some signs of hypothyroidism. For some these symptoms can be mild, but for others it can be quite significant and include exhaustion, bloating, weight gain, mood changes, and overall malaise. Of course, all these symptoms go away once the thyroid hormone replacement is restarted after the administration of the iodine, but it can be somewhat nasty during those few weeks.

One new development in the administration of radioiodine is the development of a new drug—Recombinant Human Thyrotropin (rhTSH). This new drug is sold under the brand name *Thryogen* (from a company called Genzyme) and first became available in 1998. This drug is an injection that is given in the doctor's office as two treatments a few days before the radioactive iodine treatment. This drug drives up the TSH without a prolonged period of thyroid hormone withdrawal by causing a sudden surge in TSH without the need to wait for the brain to produce lots of the hormone slowly over a few weeks. There is now considerable experience with this drug and it has been used for about seven years in many patients with thyroid cancer (Robbins, Larson et al. 2002; Elisei, Schlumberger et al. 2009). Endocrinologists prefer to have both options (thyroid hormone withdrawal or Thyrogen injection) available to them for driving up TSH. Though preliminary studies are very promising for the use of Thyrogen in many patients, there are still some patients that are probably best served with the withdrawal method. Those patients at highest risk for recurrences may benefit from thyroid hormone withdrawal because this protocol allows for a pretreatment imaging scan which helps the doctors decide the dose of radioactive iodine; whereas Thyrogen injection does not allow this imaging to be performed. The pretreatment scan does allow some dose adjustments to be made in case more metastatic sites are seen than was predicted by the physician, based on the best available data prior to treatment. One other major downside of use of Thyrogen instead of withdrawal is the added cost of using Thyrogen, which currently costs more than $1,000 per set of injections. More research is ongoing on the use of Thyrogen, but it is likely that both treatment options will remain available in the future.

If the decision is made to consider treatment with radioactive iodine, several months after total thyroidectomy for well-differentiated thyroid cancer, the patient is withdrawn from thyroid hormone and once the TSH is quite high, a diagnostic dosage of I-131 is given. This test allows physicians to see how much thyroid tissue is remaining. Frequently, even after total thyroidectomy, small amounts of thyroid tissue still remain around the recurrent laryngeal nerve and the parathyroid glands. If no remaining thyroid tissue is seen in the thyroid bed or in the lymph nodes of the neck with diagnostic amounts of I-131, the patient is considered cured and will be monitored with thyroid-stimulating hormone suppression only, which will be explained in the next section.

If any remaining thyroid tissue is seen then, an ablative dosage of radioactive iodine for treatment will be given at a subsequent visit. Timing of the second therapeutic dose is important as the diagnostic dosage of I-131 used for imaging any remaining tissue can in fact "stun" remaining thyroid tissue so that no further iodine uptake will occur (see sidebar on radioactive iodine). Patients are frequently told to eat a low iodine diet for a few weeks and then return for an ablative dosage of radioiodine to maximize its uptake. The maximum amount of radioiodine that may be given to a person outside of the hospital is 30 milicuries (mCi). Frequently, however, much larger dosages of radioactive iodine must sometimes be given in the range of 50–100 mCi and special precautions must be taken to properly dispose of the person's body fluids including sweat, saliva, and urine so that this radioactive material does not contaminate others. If even larger doses of radioactivity are used, patients must be admitted to a special portion of the hospital that has shielding to prevent radiation from spreading to other people and establish protocols to dispose of radioactive materials. Ablative dosages of radioactive iodine are absorbed into residual thyroid cells or thyroid cancer cells and then emit beta radiation, which triggers immediate cellular death.

The use of ablative radioiodine therapy is a hotly debated topic in thyroid cancer treatment. Some advocate its use and think it is associated with a reduction in the risk of recurrence of thyroid cancer by approximately 50 percent over ten years and an overall decrease in mortality rate and risk of metastases (Mazzaferri and Jhiang 1994). Others use it with more caution, citing that thyroid cancer patients have a naturally low rate of recurrence and that physicians have to be cautious about overtreatment.

It may seem counter-intuitive to treat cancer with radiation since well-differentiated thyroid cancer may be caused by radiation in the first place. However, the use of ablative dosages of radioiodine allows the destruction of any residual thyroid tissue that may be harboring thyroid cancer from the inside out. It is important to realize that radioiodine ablation is only effective for small amounts of thyroid tissue and cannot destroy an entire thyroid lobe for example. Therefore, radioiodine ablation is only suitable for patients who have received a

What History Can Teach Us:
A Collaborative Effort: The Discovery of Radioactive Iodine as a
Treatment for Hyperthyroidism
and Thyroid Cancer

Radioactive forms of iodine are now routinely used in laboratory research on the thyroid gland and aid in the diagnosis and treatment of thyroid diseases, both benign and malignant in patients. Remember that the discovery of the power of radiation and radioactivity is relatively new. In 1905, Dr. Robert Abbe had first used radium pellets sown into the thyroid gland to try to shrink it and tried Graves' disease and not long after external radiation was given as a treatment for hyperthyroidism. By 1924, Dr. George de Hevesy in Europe was working on using radioactive elements as tracers of normal minerals in the body. He later won the Nobel prize thus generating more interest in radiation and radioactive compounds. By 1934, work by the famous Madame Curie led to the ability to artificially produce many radioactive compounds for studying all kinds of physiologic processes and the thyroid gland was among the beneficiaries.

Shortly thereafter in 1936, a curious collaboration developed between doctors from the Thyroid Unit at the Massachusetts General Hospital (MGH) and scientists at The Massachusetts Institute of Technology (MIT). Dr. Karl Taylor Compton, the president of MIT had given a lecture during lunch entitled "What Physics can do for Biology and Medicine" which sparked a discussion among a group of young scientist and physicians. Over the next few years, this group (Dr. Robley Evans, Dr. Saul Hertz, Dr. James Means, and Dr. Arthur Roberts) worked feverishly on showing that radioactive iodine could be made, and if given to an animal, would be deposited and concentrated in the thyroid. Everybody realized something important and seminal was going on and their work was published (Hertz, Roberts, et al. 1940). Further work had to be done to make more of the radioactive iodine available and also to prolong its half life so it could last longer in the body. Radioactive iodine (RAI) was given for the first time to a human around 1940, and by 1941, a dose of I^{130} was given to a patient with thyroid disease. Soon thereafter other forms of RAI including the most commonly used form today I^{131} was developed. Treatment of patients with hyperthyroidism had begun and it was fairly clear from the beginning that this fascinating radioactive compound not only ended up in the thyroid but also managed to cure the patient's hyperthyroidism, getting rid of their severe symptoms without surgery or further medication. Soon enough, radioactive iodine became more widely available and made the treatment of thyrotoxicosis more practical. The physicians at the MGH then went onto study the safety and efficacy of this novel compound in treatment of various thyroid diseases including thyroid cancer. Safety comes first, so much of the early work was focused on whether the administered radioactive compound could result in toxicity, genetic mutations, and other cancers. This was the beginning of a tremendous amount of work in this arena, and radioactive iodine remains an indispensable tool for thyroid research and for treatment of patients with thyroid diseases. Remember that initial lecture given during the lunch hour more than 60 years ago? It sure did get some smart people thinking about iodine, radioactivity, and how to apply physics to the study of the thyroid gland.

total thyroidectomy. Approximately six months after receiving an ablative dosage of radioiodine, patients will then receive a follow-up whole body diagnostic scan to see how much, if any, residual thyroid tissue remains or if any metastases are present elsewhere in the body.

THYROID SUPPRESSION: USING THE BODY'S OWN FEEDBACK LOOPS

Well-differentiated thyroid cancer cells are still responsive to thyroid stimulating hormone (TSH), which causes the thyroid cancer cells to multiply in number. Therefore, following thyroid surgery, people with well-differentiated thyroid cancer are given thyroxine in sufficient dosages to suppress any TSH production by the pituitary gland. The amount of thyroxine must suppress TSH production, but not be so excessive as to cause symptoms of thyrotoxicosis including atrial fibrillation, bone loss, and anxiety among others. Again, TSH suppression is difficult to achieve if a person still has a remaining thyroid lobe and is most suitable if a person had a total thyroidectomy.

FOLLOW-UP OF WELL-DIFFERENTIATED THYROID CANCER: HOW TO LOOK FOR RECURRENCES

Patient with any kind of cancer always want to know if the doctor can tell when a cancer might be back. Recurrence, or reappearance of a cancer, can occur in some patients with well-differentiated thyroid cancers, but can often be treated and the patient still permanently cured. As mentioned previously, well-differentiated thyroid cancers continue to retain the ability to produce thyroglobulin, a specialized protein produced by thyroid follicular cells. No other cells in the body are able to make thyroglobulin. Theoretically, patients who have undergone total thryoidectomy followed by radioiodine ablation of any remnant tissue should have no living thyroid cells capable of producing thyroglobulin. Therefore, all patients who have received total thyroidectomy followed by radioiodine ablation should have a thyroglobulin level near zero. The presence of thyroglobulin levels in the blood work can serve as a marker of thyroid cancer recurrence.

Measurement of thyroglobulin levels about every six months allows physicians to detect possible recurrence of thyroid cancer very early on in the disease course. If a recurrence is detected, that person should then go for diagnostic radioiodine imaging to see where the iodine-trapping thyroid cells are hiding. This allows for possible ablation if any thyroid cancer cells are detected. Serum thyroglobulin measurements are not useful if a person still has any remaining thyroid tissue after surgery (Spencer and Wang 1995). Also unfortunately, up to 20 percent of people with thyroid cancer also have antibodies to thyroglobulin. These antibodies interfere with the chemical tests used to measure serum thyroglobulin and can result in an artificially elevated or decreased thyroglobulin level (Spencer, Takeuchi et al. 1998). Patients with interfering antibodies in their blood cannot have accurate thyroglobulin measurements performed, making this normally very useful test unusable.

During the course of monitoring for recurrent thyroid disease, some people will require repeat radioactive iodine scans. This just means that periodically doctors might want to take a look for thyroid cancer cells that might trap small doses of radioactive iodine. These tests can be done routinely in some, or more often specifically when a recurrence is suspected on recent blood work; for example if there is a sudden elevation in blood thyroglobulin levels. In order to get the best chance of maximal iodine uptake by any hidden cancer cells, the thyroid hormone suppression and any iodine supplementation is stopped so that the thyroid cancer cells become hungry for iodine. As the thyroid hormone levels drop to levels well below normal, the hypothalamic-pituitary feedback axis (see Chapter 2) kicks in and causes a massive increase in TSH. The rise in TSH causes an up regulation of the specialized iodine transporters on the surface of thyroid cancer cells. This way any recurrent thyroid cancer can take up the radioactive iodine and be seen on the radioactive iodine scans. Unfortunately, people also have many of the symptoms of hypothyroidism (see Chapter 2) and any recurrent thyroid cancer can even increase in size during the period when TSH suppression is lacking (Maloof, Vickery et al. 1956). To prevent these complications, many cancer centers now give recombinant human TSH prior to the radioactive iodine scan. Recombinant human TSH (Thyrogen, see previously) is an injectable recombinant purified version of the natural hormone TSH produced by the pituitary gland used to boost the uptake of radioactive iodine into any residual thyroid tissue or recurrent thyroid cancer without needing thyroid hormone withdrawal. Remember that some doctors use Thyrogen to boost TSH prior to the initial treatment dose of radioiodine. Here is an example where it is used to follow patients with thyroid cancer and to check for any recurrences. This is in concept based on the same principles outlined previously. The only problems with recombinant human TSH is that it is very expensive and it must be given two days in a row prior to the radioactive iodine scan. Some studies also suggest that the images obtained after recombinant TSH may not be as clear as with thyroid hormone withdrawal (Ladenson, Braverman et al. 1997).

MEDULLARY THYROID CANCERS: FASCINATING, BUT A BIT MORE FEARED

Medullary thyroid carcinomas represent approximately five percent of all thyroid malignancies. Unlike the previously mentioned well-differentiated thyroid cancers, medullary thyroid carcinomas arise from the parafollicular C-cells of the thyroid gland. As described in Chapter 2, C-cells are neural-crest derivatives and produce calcitonin. Nobody really knows what these cells normally do in the thyroid gland, but when they transform into cancerous cells, they can behave very differently than the well-differentiated thyroid cancers that are derived from the common thyroid follicular cells. Many things stand out about medullary cancer when compared to the more common papillary or follicular thyroid cancer. For one thing, about 25 percent of all medullary thyroid cancers are familial, meaning they occur because of a genetic defect or mutation within a family's lineage that makes that person susceptible to medullary thyroid cancer. Familial cases of medullary thyroid carcinoma are commonly multifocal since most, if not all, the cells in the gland contain the genetic mutation (Saad, Ordonez et al. 1984). The remaining 75 percent occur sporadically, meaning that no one else in the person's family has medullary thyroid cancer and these sporadic cases are usually limited to one side of the thyroid.

The familial medullary thyroid carcinoma syndromes are multiple endocrine neoplasia 2A (Sipple Syndrome or MEN 2A), multiple endocrine neoplasia 2B (MEN 2B), and familial medullary thyroid carcinoma. Although the names of these syndromes sound complicated, they are actually just descriptions of what other problems a person may have besides familial medullary thyroid carcinoma. People with MEN 2A have medullary thyroid carcinoma that develops in the second decade of life, combined with an adrenal gland tumor called a pheochromocytoma (in 50% of cases), and overactive parathyroid glands or hyperparathyroidism (in 10–20% of cases). People with MEN 2B have medullary thyroid carcinoma combined with pheochromocytoma (in 50% of patients), tall stature and long limbs and fingers called marfanoid habitus, and multiple tumors composed of mature nerve cells called neuromas. The form of medullary thyroid carcinoma in MEN 2B is the most aggressive of all the familial syndromes and can develop in a person as young as ten years of age. It also has a tendency for rapid growth and early metastasis to distant organs. If a person has familial medullary thyroid carcinoma only with no other types of tumors, then it is just called *familial medullary thyroid carcinoma* and typically develops during adulthood. All of the familial medullary thyroid carcinoma syndromes are autosomal dominant, which means that children inheriting a familial medullary thyroid carcinoma syndrome have a 100 percent risk of developing medullary thyroid cancer. Therefore all people with medullary thyroid carcinoma should undergo genetic testing to determine if the etiology of their carcinoma is familial or sporadic (Jimenez, Hu et al. 2008). It is important to figure out if a particular patient has this syndrome since if a pheochromocytoma is present it should be found prior to the thyroid surgery. Because pheochromocytomas while usually benign, can be life threatening as it can secrete excessive amounts of adrenaline (epinephrine) or noradrenaline (norepinephrine).

The diagnosis of medullary thyroid carcinoma is very similar to well-differentiated thyroid carcinoma in terms of fine-needle aspiration biopsy and neck ultrasound. Medullary cancer though does have a much higher chance of getting out of the thyroid and metastasizing to nearby lymph nodes then spreading to other parts of the body. This can happen even when the medullary cancer inside the thyroid itself is quite small. Once diagnosed, medullary thyroid carcinoma should be treated with total thyroidectomy and lymphadenectomy of any involved compartments of the neck. Usually many more lymph nodes are removed from the areas surrounding the thyroid, since these lymph nodes are often harboring metastatic medullary cancer cells. Post-operatively, since medullary thyroid cancer cells are not derived from thyroid follicular cells, they do not have specialized iodine receptors and thus does not take up radioiodine. Therefore radioiodine imaging and ablation are not effective therapeutic tools against medullary thyroid cancer. If residual or recurrent medullary thyroid cancer is suspected, surgery can often be repeated to remove any additional foci of disease. If surgery is not possible or the tumor has spread, external beam radiation treatments, chemotherapy, or specialized targeted therapies may be useful in slowing cancer progression (see Chapter 8) (Shimaoka, Schoenfeld et al. 1985).

PRIMARY THYROID LYMPHOMA: A RARE BIRD

Thyroid lymphoma is one of the least common thyroid cancers and predominantly occurs in people in the fifth to eighth decades of life. Thyroid lymphoma is really a cancer of the white blood cells that happens to be found inside the thyroid gland. Almost all people with thyroid lymphoma also have chronic lymphocytic thyroiditis (Hashimoto's disease). Remember that in Hashimoto's thyroiditis, the body attacks the thyroid with antibodies and white blood immune cells. These same immune cells live in the thyroid in large numbers, and in some patients, the white blood cells themselves can sometimes become cancerous while residing in the thyroid tissue. Many different types of lymphoma have been reported, but the most common type of thyroid lymphoma is non-Hodgkin's B-cell tumors such as diffuse large-cell lymphoma (Skarsgard, Connors et al. 1991). Fine-needle biopsies of thyroid lymphoma typically reveal sheets of lymphoid cells that may be difficult to distinguish from anaplastic thyroid cancer. All people who may have thyroid lymphoma should receive a computed tomographic scan of the brain, neck, chest, abdomen, and pelvis and a bone-marrow biopsy to evaluate for any other sources of lymphoma. Thyroid lymphoma is very sensitive to external radiation. Most of the time, thyroid lymphoma is treated like lymphoma anywhere else in the body with chemotherapy and radiation. Rarely, thyroid lymphoma that is small and limited to the thyroid gland is treated with total thyroidectomy followed by post-operative radiation therapy. This treatment results in a five-year survival rate of up to 85 percent (Pyke, Grant et al. 1992). The presence of lymphoma outside of the thyroid gland has a greatly reduced five-year survival rate of less than 35 percent (Junor, Paul et al. 1992).

ANAPLASTIC THYROID CANCER: THE WORST ONE YET

Anaplastic thyroid carcinoma is also a very uncommon thyroid malignancy and accounts for only one to two percent of all thyroid cancers in the United States (Hundahl, Fleming et al. 1998). Unfortunately, it is also the most aggressive thyroid cancer and has the worst prognosis. Unlike, well-differentiated thyroid cancer cells, anaplastic thyroid cancer cells exist purely to consume limited resources and rapidly reproduce. Of all the thyroid cancers, anaplastic thyroid carcinoma presents the latest in life typically in the sixth or seventh decade of life (Are and Shaha 2006). Anaplastic thyroid carcinoma grows very rapidly and spreads through direct invasion of surrounding structures. These structures include the trachea and/or recurrent laryngeal nerve, and also the esophagus, jugular veins, and carotid arteries. Unfortunately, anaplastic thyroid carcinoma also forms metastases early on, and 50–60 percent of people with anaplastic thyroid carcinoma already have distant metastases to lungs, bone, and brain at the time of diagnosis (Tennvall, Lundell et al. 2002). People with anaplastic thyroid cancer often present to their physician with a rapidly growing hard neck mass that seems attached to other structures in the neck, hoarseness, and/or difficulty swallowing (Giuffrida and Gharib 2000). The diagnosis is typically from fine-needle aspiration biopsy, and if diagnosed early, the treatment of anaplastic thyroid cancer is total thyroidectomy as well as any other structures involved. Resection is not possible in the majority of people with anaplastic thyroid cancer. Sometimes patients are given a *tracheostomy* or breathing hole in their neck so that the cancer does not obstruct their airway as it grows. Unfortunately, anaplastic thyroid cancer cells do not take up iodine or most chemotheraputic agents and are resistant to external radiation. Most patents with anaplastic thyroid cancer die within six months of diagnosis due to extensive lung metastases, airway obstruction, tumor related bleeding, or heart failure (Kitamura, Shimizu et al. 1999). Some experimental therapies are being developed for anaplastic thyroid cancer and will be discussed in Chapter 8.

REFERENCES

Agency, I. A. E. (2006). Environmental consequences of the Chernobyl accident and their remediation: Twenty years of experience. Report of the Chernobyl Forum Expert Group Environment. International Atomic Energy Agency. Vienna.

Altekruse, S. F., K. C., Krapcho M., et al. (May 5, 2010). "*SEER Cancer Statistics Review, 1975–2007.*" Retrieved May 5, 2010, from http://seer.cancer.gov/csr/1975_2007/.

Are, C. and A. R. Shaha (2006). "Anaplastic thyroid carcinoma: biology, pathogenesis, prognostic factors, and treatment approaches." *Ann Surg Oncol* **13**(4): 453–64.

Boice, J. D., Jr. and J. H. Lubin (1997). "Occupational and environmental radiation and cancer." *Cancer Causes Control* **8**(3): 309–22.

Chen, A. Y., A. Jemal, et al. (2009). "Increasing incidence of differentiated thyroid cancer in the United States, 1988–2005." *Cancer* **115**(16): 3801–7.

Davies, L. and H. G. Welch (2006). "Increasing incidence of thyroid cancer in the United States, 1973–2002." *JAMA* **295**(18): 2164–67.

De Cort M, D. G., Fridman Sh. D., et al. (1998). Atlas of caesium deposition on Europe after the Chernobyl accident. European Commission Report 16733. Luxembourg.

DeGroot, L. J., E. L. Kaplan, et al. (1990). "Natural history, treatment, and course of papillary thyroid carcinoma." *J Clin Endocrinol Metab* **71**(2): 414–24.

Elisei, R., M. Schlumberger, et al. (2009). "Follow-up of low-risk differentiated thyroid cancer patients who underwent radioiodine ablation of postsurgical thyroid remnants after either recombinant human thyrotropin or thyroid hormone withdrawal." *J Clin Endocrinol Metab* **94**(11): 4171–79.

Enewold, L., K. Zhu, et al. (2009). "Rising thyroid cancer incidence in the United States by demographic and tumor characteristics, 1980–2005." *Cancer Epidemiol Biomarkers Prev* **18**(3): 784–91.

Engeland, A., S. Tretli, et al. (2006). "Body size and thyroid cancer in two million Norwegian men and women." *Br J Cancer* **95**(3): 366–70.

Ezzat, S., D. A. Sarti, et al. (1994). "Thyroid incidentalomas. Prevalence by palpation and ultrasonography." *Arch Intern Med* **154**(16): 1838–40.

Giuffrida, D. and H. Gharib (2000). "Anaplastic thyroid carcinoma: current diagnosis and treatment." *Ann Oncol* **11**(9): 1083–89.

Goodman, M. T., L. N. Kolonel, et al. (1992). "The association of body size, reproductive factors and thyroid cancer." *Br J Cancer* **66**(6): 1180–84.

Grebe, S. K. and I. D. Hay (1995). "Follicular thyroid cancer." *Endocrinol Metab Clin North Am* **24**(4): 761–801.

Hannibal, C. G., A. Jensen, et al. (2008). "Risk of thyroid cancer after exposure to fertility drugs: results from a large Danish cohort study." *Hum Reprod* **23**(2): 451–56.

Hegedus, L. (2004). "Clinical practice. The thyroid nodule." *N Engl J Med* **351**(17): 1764–71.

Hertz, S., J. H. Means, et al. (1940). "Radioactive iodine as an indicator in thyroid physiology: iodine collection by normal and hyperplastic thyroids in rabbits." *Am J Physiol* **128**: 565–76.

Hundahl, S. A., B. Cady, et al. (2000). "Initial results from a prospective cohort study of 5583 cases of thyroid carcinoma treated in the United States during 1996. U.S. and German Thyroid Cancer Study Group. An American College of Surgeons Commission on Cancer Patient Care Evaluation study." *Cancer* **89**(1): 202–17.

Hundahl, S. A., I. D. Fleming, et al. (1998). "A National Cancer Data Base report on 53,856 cases of thyroid carcinoma treated in the U.S., 1985–1995 [see comments]." *Cancer* **83**(12): 2638–48.

Jacob, P., T. I. Bogdanova, et al. (2006). "Thyroid cancer risk in areas of Ukraine and Belarus affected by the Chernobyl accident." *Radiat Res* **165**(1): 1–8.

Jimenez, C., M. I. Hu, et al. (2008). "Management of medullary thyroid carcinoma." *Endocrinol Metab Clin North Am* **37**(2): 481–96, x–xi.

Junor, E. J., J. Paul, et al. (1992). "Primary non-Hodgkin's lymphoma of the thyroid." *Eur J Surg Oncol* **18**(4): 313–21.

Kitamura, Y., K. Shimizu, et al. (1999). "Immediate causes of death in thyroid carcinoma: clinicopathological analysis of 161 fatal cases." *J Clin Endocrinol Metab* **84**(11): 4043–49.

Ladenson, P. W., L. E. Braverman, et al. (1997). "Comparison of administration of recombinant human thyrotropin with withdrawal of thyroid hormone for radioactive iodine scanning in patients with thyroid carcinoma." *N Engl J Med* **337**(13): 888–96.

Maloof, F., A. L. Vickery, et al. (1956). "An evaluation of various factors influencing the treatment of metastatic thyroid carcinoma with I 131." *J Clin Endocrinol Metab* **16** (1): 1–27.

Mazzaferri, E. L., G. M. Doherty, et al. (2009). "The pros and cons of prophylactic central compartment lymph node dissection for papillary thyroid carcinoma." *Thyroid* **19**(7): 683–89.

Mazzaferri, E. L. and S. M. Jhiang (1994). "Long-term impact of initial surgical and medical therapy on papillary and follicular thyroid cancer." *Am J Med* **97**(5): 418–28.

McHenry, C. R. and B. A. Sandoval (1998). "Management of follicular and Hurthle cell neoplasms of the thyroid gland." *Surg Oncol Clin N Am* **7**(4): 893–910.

Pyke, C. M., C. S. Grant, et al. (1992). "Non-Hodgkin's lymphoma of the thyroid: is more than biopsy necessary?" *World J Surg* **16**(4): 604–9; discussion 609–10.

Rezzonico, J., M. Rezzonico, et al. (2008). "Introducing the thyroid gland as another victim of the insulin resistance syndrome." *Thyroid* **18**(4): 461–64.

Richards, M. L., E. Bohnenblust, et al. (2008). "Nondiagnostic thyroid fine-needle aspiration biopsies are no longer a dilemma." *Am J Surg* **196**(3): 398–402.

Robbins, R. J., S. M. Larson, et al. (2002). "A retrospective review of the effectiveness of recombinant human TSH as a preparation for radioiodine thyroid remnant ablation." *J Nucl Med* **43**(11): 1482–88.

Saad, M. F., N. G. Ordonez, et al. (1984). "Medullary carcinoma of the thyroid. A study of the clinical features and prognostic factors in 161 patients." *Medicine* (Baltimore) **63** (6): 319–42.

Schlinkert, R. T., J. A. van Heerden, et al. (1997). "Factors that predict malignant thyroid lesions when fine-needle aspiration is 'suspicious for follicular neoplasm.'" *Mayo Clin Proc* 72(10): 913–16.

Schneider, A. B. and D. H. Sarne (2005). "Long-term risks for thyroid cancer and other neoplasms after exposure to radiation." *Nat Clin Pract Endocrinol Metab* 1(2): 82–91.

Shimaoka, K., D. A. Schoenfeld, et al. (1985). "A randomized trial of doxorubicin versus doxorubicin plus cisplatin in patients with advanced thyroid carcinoma." *Cancer* 56 (9): 2155–60.

Skarsgard, E. D., J. M. Connors, et al. (1991). "A current analysis of primary lymphoma of the thyroid." *Arch Surg* 126(10): 1199–203; discussion 1203–4.

Spencer, C. A., M. Takeuchi, et al. (1998). "Serum thyroglobulin autoantibodies: prevalence, influence on serum thyroglobulin measurement, and prognostic significance in patients with differentiated thyroid carcinoma." *J Clin Endocrinol Metab* 83(4): 1121–27.

Spencer, C. A. and C. C. Wang (1995). "Thyroglobulin measurement. Techniques, clinical benefits, and pitfalls." *Endocrinol Metab Clin North Am* 24(4): 841–63.

Tennvall, J., G. Lundell, et al. (2002). "Anaplastic thyroid carcinoma: three protocols combining doxorubicin, hyperfractionated radiotherapy and surgery." *Br J Cancer* 86(12): 1848–53.

6

Thyroid Surgery

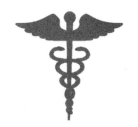

Surgeons are given a large responsibility by society. No other profession is allowed to cut into the human body, manipulate the body parts, and hope things turn out for the better, that the disease is cured or at least kept at bay. Surgeons of previous centuries had a harder job to do, certainly with much less detailed understanding of anatomy and physiology and little in the ways of anesthetics or aseptic techniques so essential to the practice of modern surgery. Surgery on the thyroid gland essentially delineates step-by-step the evolution of modern surgery. Indeed it is clear that as the knowledge of what the function of the thyroid was developed as brave surgeons were slowly but surely understanding the steps required to safely operate on or remove this organ.

THE EARLY HISTORY OF THYROID SURGERY: NEARLY ALWAYS A DEATH SENTENCE

The history of thyroid surgery really starts when physicians in the ancient times recognized goiter as a distinct entity. Remember from the first chapter that goiter is basically an enlargement of the thyroid, sometimes mild, other times quite massive. Goiters are documented as early as 600 AD in Chinese medical texts, and it is in approximately 500 AD that a surgeon in Baghdad (modern day Iraq) was documented to *excise* (surgically remove) a thyroid goiter—a feat that led to massive blood loss and almost killed the patient. Over the ensuing 1,000 years, physicians and surgeons used various means of controlling an enlarged thyroid, some were treated with special salves or ointments meant to reduce the size, others were *ligated* (tied up or bound up using something like a surgical string) using ropes or shoestrings, the pressure caused by the strangling of the tissue in between the tight ligature results in *necrosis* of the gland (necrosis is when part of a tissue or organ dies). Unfortunately most of these therapies only led to temporary improvement in some, and a worse fate in most with infection, *sepsis*, (otherwise known as blood poisoning when bacteria or toxins enter the bloodstream, often causing death.

During the Italian Renaissance, much emphasis was placed on understanding human anatomy, including seminal work by Leonardo da Vinci who described the thyroid as two globular sack-like glands in the neck, though he did not speculate on the functional nature of the gland. Later in the seventeenth century, the gland was named *glandulam thyroideam*, which in Latin means the shape of a shield, which is of course how the two lobes of the thyroid looked to the anatomist of that time.

Remarkably, the first thyroid surgery using scalpels to cut out the organ was performed in 1646 by Fabricus. Things did not end well for either the ten-year-old patient who died, nor for the surgeon who was quickly imprisoned. It took another 150 years before European surgeons tried the surgery again. In 1791, Pierre-Joseph Desault performed a successful *partial thyroidectomy* where he removed half the organ, and in 1808, Guillaume Dupuytren performed the first *total thyroidectomy*, removing the entire thyroid gland. By the 1850s, surgery on the thyroid gland had become more commonplaces with surgeons across Europe dabbling in it (Halsted 1920). *Mortality* (death) rates from any kind of attempted thyroid surgery remained astronomically high, with pretty much 40 percent of patients dying after thyroid surgery. One thing surgeons understood fairly quickly about surgery on this gland was the impressive blood supply to the gland, especially when enlarged. This large amount of blood flowing into this gland made things very tricky for early surgeons. Remember that they had none of the modern tools with which to stop bleeding. Pressure on the bleeding vessels, and suture material to form surgical ties around larger vessels were all that was available in that period. In fact, thyroid surgery was thought to be so dangerous, that in 1866, the famous American surgeon Dr. Samuel David Gross noted, "Can the thyroid gland . . . be removed with a reasonable hope of saving the patient? Experience emphatically answers NO. . . . If a surgeon should be so foolhardy as to undertake it . . . every stroke of the knife will be followed by a torrent of blood, and lucky will it be for him if his victim lives long enough to enable him to finish his horrid butchery. No honest and sensible surgeon would ever engage in it" (Shields 1999).

THE EVOLUTION OF MODERN THYROID SURGERY: DRAMATIC CHANGES FOR THE BETTER

The advancement of modern day surgery in general, and thyroid surgery specifically as we know it today, mostly grew out of two remarkable advances:

1. The ability to administer safe *anesthesia* (induced loss of sensitivity to pain and sometimes unconsciousness) to patients undergoing surgery.
2. The introduction of sterile surgical techniques and antisepsis.

With the advent of anesthetics, surgeons could take their time, study their techniques, and slowly make changes that gradually transformed thyroid surgery from a form of "butchery" to one of the safest surgical procedures performed today. In 1846, Dr. William Morton at the Massachusetts General Hospital demonstrated that a new drug called Ether could be used to anesthetize a patient safely during a surgical procedure by Dr. John Collins Warren, rendering them unconscious and pain free (Toledo 2006). Around the same time, Joseph Lister introduced the concept that sterility was important to safe surgery (Herr 2007). Prior to Lister's work, surgeons didn't use gloves, did not wash their instruments, and made no extra efforts to keep the procedure even remotely clean. Lister and a whole crew of physician scientist introduced sterility into the operative room along with steam sterilization of the actual instruments used by the surgeons. Think of that, so different from how we see surgeons today wearing scrubs, sterile gowns, masks, hair bonnets, and sterile gloves using sterile instruments in a sterilized field. Once the importance of sterility and the proper administration of anesthesia were firmly accepted by surgeons in Europe and the United States, some additional tweaking with improved instruments made for *hemostasis* (stopping bleeding), thyroid surgery was primed and ready for major changes.

Two surgeons are credited with the development of modern thyroid surgery: Albert Theodor Bilroth who worked tirelessly on a variety of surgical techniques first in Zurich and then in Vienna. He described techniques for thyroid surgery in his books and was an influential teacher of surgery. However, Theodor Kocher is undoubtedly the father of modern day thyroid surgery. Kocher worked in Switzerland, not only on developing the meticulous techniques used in thyroid surgery today, but also on the physiology and pathology of this complex endocrine organ. During his active years, he operated on thousands of patients with thyroid disease and ultimately managed to reduce the mortality from 13 percent in the 1870s to 0.2 percent in 1898. His remarkable work did not go unnoticed and resulted in him becoming the first surgeon to win the prestigious Nobel Prize in Medicine and Physiology.

What History Can Teach Us
Emil Theodor Kocher: The First Surgeon to Win a Nobel Prize

There is no more prestigious prize than the annual Nobel Prize given for out-standing achievements in chemistry, physics, medicine, literature, and for works in peace. The Nobel Prize in Medicine and Physiology has been given to the best and the brightest medical minds in Europe since its inception in 1901. However, this important prize had never been given to a surgeon before 1909, when this great honor was bestowed upon Emil Theodor Kocher, a Swiss surgeon who contributed immensely not only to the safety of thyroid surgery as we know it today, but also to a much deeper understanding of the anatomy and physiology of the thyroid gland. Thyroid goiter was a big problem in Europe since iodine in food was scarce (iodination of salt did not become customary until much later). Very large goiters of the kind rarely seen today in Europe were very common. Patients who had to undergo thyroid surgery of any kind were in mortal danger. That statement is no exaggeration since almost half the patients who had thyroid operations died. This all changed through the systematic and thoughtful efforts of Kocher. Before Kocher, the thyroid had been described, studied, and even removed but its function was not known. Nobody before Kocher had understood that the thyroid produced a hormone that was essential to most key functions in the human body, from the skin to muscle function to brain power. In 1867, Kocher made a keen observation in one of his patients—an 11-year-girl named Marie Bishel who had to have the entire thyroid removed (McGreevy and Miller 1969). The child's normal development had slowed, including significant short stature and the child had become shorter than younger siblings, and had developed swollen hands, a puffy face and a had remarkable decrease in intelligence. This sudden realization made Kocher go back and analyze all the patients he had performed thyroidectomies on and soon he realized that removing the thyroid led to some kind of deficiency which he initially called "cachexi strumipriva" and later called *cachexia thyreopriv*; known today as *hypothyroidism*. He had noticed for the first time what happens to humans, and especially children, if they lack thyroid hormone for a long period of time. He then pursued the study of the physiology and pathology of the thyroid gland with passion even though he was a surgeon first and foremost.

He went on to develop and recommend a safe form of thyroid surgery where in some patients a small piece of thyroid tissue was left behind instead of removal of the entire thyroid gland (*subtotal thyroidectomy*). For those who needed to have surgical removal of the entire thyroid, he introduced oral replacement therapy with administration of *"thyroid juice"* (*Nobel Foundation 2010*) to patients in whom the whole thyroid was removed. When he started his study of the thyroid gland in 1870, mortality rates for thyroidectomy were 40 percent, and in just a few short years, he managed to drop the mortality rates to less than one percent. He became famous in Europe as the "go to surgeon," and by 1917, when he died, he had performed more than 7,000 thyroidectomies. Surgeons came from all over the world to learn his techniques. His book *Erkrankungen der Schilddrüse* (*Diseases of the thyroid gland*) was an in depth review of the symptoms and treatment strategies for thyroid diseases. His new ideas on the physiology and pathology of the thyroid gland caused controversy at that time, but in fact, surgeons today still use many of the instruments and techniques that Kocher described over 100 years ago. Kocher was a remarkable surgeon and had immense contribution to many areas of surgery, including the concept of antiseptics and sterility which is now a cornerstone of modern surgery, hernia surgery, surgery on the stomach and intestines. However, it was his major discoveries about the pathology, physiology, and surgery of the thyroid gland won him the Nobel Prize in Medicine in 1909, a remarkable feat for a surgeon then and now.

The European surgeons who had trained with Bilroth made one other discovery critical to safe thyroid surgery. In the late 1880s, it was already known that some patients undergoing total thyroidectomy went on to develop severe muscular *tetany* (severe cramping of the muscles throughout the body); in some cases, this postoperative tetany lead to death since the heart is also a muscle and a "cramped" heart is not a good thing. In 1891, Dr. Eugene Emile Gley attributed this strange post-operative complication to the removal of tiny glands that shared a blood supply with the thyroid gland called parathyroid glands. The parathyroid glands which are the size of lentils in humans had first been discovered in 1850 by anatomist Richard Owen while performing an autopsy on a rhinoceros in the London Zoo and was later also found in dogs by a medical student Ivar Sandstrom. In the late 1880s, Sandstrom described important anatomic details about the 4 parathyroids in 50 human *cadavers* (a dissected dead body), including important discoveries about their variability, anatomical position, location. By early in the twentieth century, it had become clear that tetany caused by removal of the parathyroids could be fixed in animals by giving parathyroid extract. Shortly thereafter, it became clear that these glands had something to do with calcium metabolism and when they were removed or damaged inadvertently during thyroid surgery, low calcium resulted and led to impressive tetany. It was not until the late 1960s that physiology of the parathyroid glands were detailed by Drs. Soloman and Berson and Rosalyn Sussman Yalow, work for which they also earned a Nobel Prize in Medicine and Physiology.

Once Kocher's techniques of thyroid surgery had been established in Europe, it was Dr. William Halsted who went for training in Europe and is credited for bringing back these surgical techniques to the United States. In the United States, Halsted helped establish the first surgical residency at Johns Hopkins Hospital in Baltimore. There he trained many American surgeons who then went

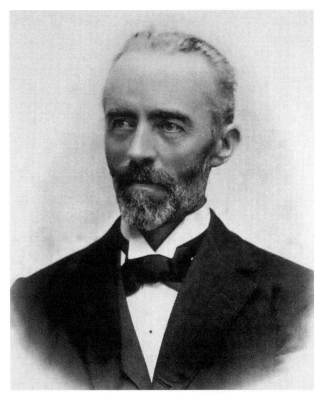

Emil Theodor Kocher (1841–1917) was a Swiss surgeon who published numerous articles about thyroid physiology and how to safely remove the thyroid gland surgically. He was the first surgeon to win the Nobel Prize in Medicine and Physiology in 1909 for his tremendous contributions to the care of patients with thyroid diseases. (National Library of Medicine)

onto illustrious careers across the United States including the establishment of the Mayo Clinic in Minnesota and the Lahey Clinic outside of Boston where additional refinements in thyroid surgery ensued. The importance of taking extra care around the recurrent laryngeal nerves, which supply movement to the vocal cords, was firmly emphasized by Dr. Frank Howard Lahey in the 1930s and 1940s. It became clear from the work of Kocher, who recommended if at all possible, leave the posterior portion of the thyroid gland behind to keep the voice as normal as possible. In Lahey's important work 30 years later, he stressed that maintaining the integrity of these paired nerves coming directly out of the brain (central nerves), was critical to retaining normal function of the vocal cords (Lahey and Hoover 1938).

Surgeons today owe their safe surgical techniques to the amazing feats of each of these surgeons and many others who put together the pieces of the puzzle that had led to the remarkable safety of thyroid surgery today. Surgeons today decide whether to perform a partial thyroidectomy or a total thyroidectomy for a variety of thyroid diseases knowing that the hard work of their predecessors has made their patients safe. Surgeons today work with well-trained anesthesiologists, impressive tools for hemostasis, and a large array of sterile instruments and assistants. Thyroid surgery in the United States is often performed by general surgeons who often have extra training in endocrine surgery or ear, nose, and throat surgeons who have become super-specialized in thyroid surgery.

DIFFERENT TYPES OF THYROID SURGERY: HALF OR WHOLE BASICALLY SAYS IT ALL

The most common reason for thyroid surgery is the presence of abnormal growths or nodules, in the thyroid. Thyroid nodules are essentially lumps found in the thyroid gland and can vary in size from several millimeters to many centimeters (see Chapter 4 for details on thyroid nodules and thyroid goiter). Very large nodules may replace nearly half the thyroid and are visible to the naked eye. Very small thyroid nodules detected only on a neck ultrasound are unlikely to be of any clinical significance. Sometimes, these nodules can be cancerous and the most common thyroid cancer seen is papillary thyroid cancer. Not every patient with thyroid nodules needs surgery. The decision to operate is made after careful consideration of the patient's history and the results of tests that have been done to evaluate the nodules and the functioning of the thyroid gland. There are several different procedures that may be done during thyroid surgery, as listed here. Once the decision for thyroid surgery has been made, the type of procedure surgeons choose depends on a number of factors: the patient's age and gender, size of the nodule in the thyroid, location of the nodule, results of fine needle aspiration, existence of enlarged lymph nodes in the neck, or a history of radiation. Surgeons decide with input from the patient and their endocrinologist which procedure is best suited to each patient's problem. Three kinds of thyroid surgery are commonly used and are listed here:

Thyroid lobectomy: One half of the thyroid is removed
Total thyroidectomy: The entire thyroid gland is removed
Lymph node dissection: Removal of some of some lymph nodes around the thyroid gland

For all thyroid operations, the incision is placed in the lower neck along the collar line, preferably in an existing skin crease or wrinkle. In general

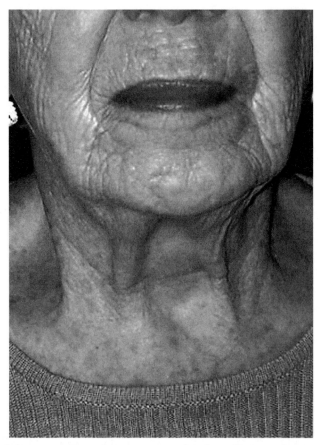

A well-healed postoperative incision one year after thyroid surgery. Incisions are often quite cosmetically pleasing, especially if hidden in a wrinkle as seen here. (Courtesy of Dr. Sareh Parangi, MD)

thyroidectomy incisions are between four and eight centimeters in length. Most surgeons perform thyroidectomies under general anesthesia with the help of an anesthesiologist. A few surgeons report safe operations with local anes-thesia and intravenous sedation with an anesthesiologist present (Spanknebel, Chabot et al. 2005). Patients have a chance prior to the operation to meet the anesthesiologist and go over details about the anesthetic plan and which type of anesthesia may be used. Just before the operation they are introduced to the whole surgical team, nurses, surgical assistants, surgical technicians, nurse anesthetists, surgical residents, and the anesthesiologist. Getting to know the whole team is important for patients since trust in your surgical team helps patients do better.

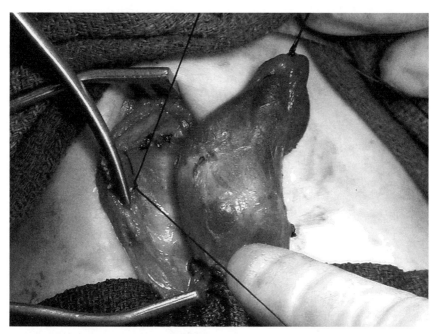

An intraoperative photograph of a left thyroid lobectomy. The left thyroid lobe is separated from the right lobe using a metal clamp and tied with a suture. The whitish structure beneath the thyroid gland is the trachea or windpipe. (Courtesy of Dr. Sareh Parangi, MD)

Thyroid Lobectomy (Partial Thyroidectomy)

The most minimal thyroid operation is a thyroid lobectomy where one half of the thyroid is removed. Patients who have half their thyroid removed usually do not need to take any thyroid hormone post-surgery. This operation is often done if the diagnosis is not clearly a cancer after the fine needle aspiration. During a partial thyroidectomy, the blood vessels to that part of the thyroid are divided, the recurrent laryngeal nerve is identified up to the voice box, and the parathyroid glands on that side are left alone, if possible. Finding and preserving the nerve to the voice box is the most arduous and difficult part of the procedure as the nerve is often quite stuck to the back of the thyroid as it sits in a tight thick band of tissue called the Ligament of Berry. Once the removed thyroid tissue is handed to the pathologist, a determination is made whether the tissue is cancerous. If the thyroid tissue is deemed cancerous during the operation, the other half of the thyroid is removed. The pathologist often cannot make the diagnosis of cancer during the operation, and they will need to look at the tissue sections under the microscope once fully processed a few days to a week later. It may be necessary to perform a second operation a few days later to remove the remainder of the thyroid gland.

Total Thyroidectomy (Complete Thyroidectomy)

A total thyroidectomy involves removal of the entire thyroid gland. This operation is performed if the fine needle aspiration shows a definite thyroid cancer or if there are multiple abnormalities in the thyroid gland. A total thyroidectomy may be considered when thyroid cancer is highly suspected or there are additional risk factors such as radiation exposure. Some cases of benign thyroid disease, such as thyroiditis or Graves' disease, are also treated with total thyroidectomy. When patients are contemplating this procedure, they should consider the post-surgery need for lifelong thyroid hormone replacement. While five percent of patients having a partial thyroidectomy may need to take thyroid hormone replacement, all patients having a total thyroidectomy take thyroid hormone pills for the rest of their life.

Lymph Node Dissection (Limited or Modified Radical)

Lymph node dissection is needed if the thyroid gland contains a papillary or follicular cancer and there are enlarged or hard lymph nodes (see Chapter 5). Most surgeons in the United States remove only the involved lymph nodes and not every last lymph node in the area. The major risks of removal of some lymph nodes are: a longer scar in some cases and injury to important nerves that include the spinal accessory nerve which could result in shoulder weakness.

RISKS OF THYROID SURGERY: EXPERIENCE COUNTS FOR SOMETHING

The risk factors listed below are possible complications that may occur with surgery. In general, the chance of complication is increased with total thyroidectomies or anytime a second or third operation is being done in the same area. Surgeons spend a lot of time talking to their patients about these possible risks of thyroid surgery. Surgeons and patients both wish that thyroid surgery could be performed with no risk and little or no scarring on the skin. Alas, this is not possible; there are still a small number of patients who end up with sometimes serious lifelong complications from thyroid surgery. It is important for patients to have trust in their surgeons, experience and proper training count a lot towards reducing these risks.

Permanent injury to the recurrent laryngeal nerve (1–2%), this can result in hoarseness or a "breathy" voice. If this complication occurs, the voice quality often adjusts with time. If no improvement is seen after two months, the vocal cord on the injured site can undergo treatments to help gain a more natural voice.

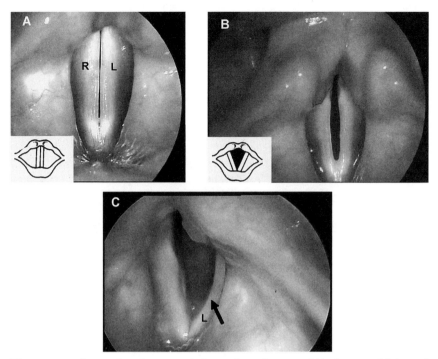

The nerves to the vocal cords are at risk during thyroid surgery. (A), the normal left vocal cord is marked with an L and the normal right vocal cord with an R. With phonation the normal vocal cords are oscillate back and forth symmetrically (B). The left recurrent laryngeal nerve is injured and the left vocal cord is bowed and not functioning normally (C, white arrow). Nerve paralysis changes the way air passes through the vocal cords and can result in a hoarse or whispery voice in some people. (Courtesy Dr. James Burns, MD)

Injury to the external branch of the superior laryngeal nerve, a small nerve important to singers. This can lead to voice fatigue, and some difficulty with high tones.

Injury to one or more of the parathyroid glands important in regulation of the calcium in the blood. Following total thyroidectomy, some patients may experience numbness and tingling in the finger tips or around their mouth. This is treated with increased intake of calcium and vitamin D. Most injuries to the parathyroid glands are temporary, only two percent of patients have permanent injury to the parathyroids. In case of permanent injury, the patient will have to take calcium and vitamin D supplements.

Very rarely bleeding in the neck occurs and may need an emergency re-operation.

One More Thing to Know: Now That's Interesting But Don't Try This at Home: Imagine You Are the Surgeon: The ABCs of Thyroid Surgery

How do surgeons learn thyroid surgery? It all looks so easy and glamorous on TV. This is not easy stuff and it takes years to master but every surgeon learns to break down operations into steps, much like cooking. They follow the steps of the operation, being careful about every step and making sure to only move on once they are secure that the last step went just fine. It is a combination of skill and art, not very different than cooking. Becoming an excellent cook can takes years to master and so can surgery. Thyroid surgery provides an excellent example of an operation where the surgeon needs to not only understand completely the detailed preoperative work-up algorithms needed, but needs to integrate this knowledge with intricate anatomic detail and surgical technical skill. Surgeons know that proper knot tying techniques will be absolutely necessary for this operation, the small thyroidal vessels do not allow for undue tension created by the inexperienced knot tier, thus finesse in knot tying is important. Surgeons find thyroid surgery not only to be gratifying in multiple levels but will also find that thyroid surgery will push their technical skill and knowledge to its limit. Before starting any operations, surgeons must know the details of the thyroidal vascular and pertinent neuroanatomical natural variants for the external branch of the superior laryngeal nerve, recurrent laryngeal nerve, and thyroidal vessels. Of course, every surgeon will have small differences in their preferences, and each one comes up with their own unique way of doing things.

Surgery is like a team sport, you have to have a competent team. But here is a glimpse of all the steps a typical thyroid surgeon takes to successfully complete a thyroid operation to remove half the thyroid (partial thyroidectomy).

1. The surgeon brings to the operating room critical knowledge of preoperative work up of the patient being operated on that day:
   a. Remember that the surgeon comes into the operating room having intimate knowledge of the patient's past medical history and thyroid condition, the reason for operation, size and side of any nodules, and the thyroid function status of the patient. Previous neck operations and whether those operations caused any problems with the function of the vocal cord or parathyroid glands have been noted. The surgeon understands how the patient's thyroid condition manifested, what work up was done, and why the decision was made to bring the patient to the operating room.
   b. Imaging studies such as ultrasounds are reviewed.
   c. The surgeon discusses the operation being undertaken and answers any last minute questions the patient may have about the operation, complications, or anticipated recovery.
   d. The surgeon communicates clearly with the anesthesia staff any concerns about anticipated problems with the patient's airway or anesthetics. The surgeon will discuss with the anesthesiologist whether muscle relaxation

should be used (especially if recurrent laryngeal nerve monitoring is being used).

2. The surgeon marks the patient's neck:

   a. The patient's neck should be marked preoperatively along natural skin creases if possible while sitting up. Even if natural skin creases cannot be used for incision placement, they can be used as a template for the incision the surgeon makes. Because asymmetric incisions draw more attention to themselves, all thyroid incisions need to be symmetric (even if only one side of the thyroid is being removed).

3. The surgeon keeps a careful eye on the neck and airway as the anesthesiologist puts the patient to sleep under anesthesia.

4. The surgeon helps the nurses and anesthesiologist position the patient on the operating room table:

   a. The patient is positioned with a shoulder roll, placed horizontally or vertically in between the shoulder blades. A small puffy bag or small roll is ideal. The head is then hyperextended and well supported using a special pillow. The head of the bed is then moved placed higher than the body. The surgeon makes sure both arms are tucked by the side and well padded.

   b. The surgeon often wears special magnification glasses called surgical loupes and a headlight given the small surgical field and to help with magnification.

5. The surgeon starts the operation

   a. A surgical time out is taken to identify the patient, and make sure the correct operation is being done on the correct patient and that all the team members agree. There is a last minute check of all the equipment necessary to perform the surgery.

   b. A transverse incision following a natural crease if possible is made by the surgeon paying attention to maintaining symmetry using the chin and sternal notch marks as midline. Incision sizes vary (often 3–8 cm) but in general the smallest size incision that makes a safe operation possible is used.

   c. This operation requires finesse and attention to performing every move delicately. Due to the fact that surgical loupes are used and the operative field is small the surgeon must remain focused on the surgical field which means the nurses or operating room technicians have to be very careful and deliberate about handing the surgeon instruments without causing distraction.

   d. In all thyroid operations (total or partial thyroidectomy), the thin muscles of the neck called the platysma are pulled away from the underlying structures superiorly and inferiorly.

   e. Once the surgeon gets to the deeper layers, two strap muscles, the sternohyoid muscle, and the sternothyroid muscle more posteriorly are separated and retracted laterally to allow visualization of the thyroid. Since the incision size is small, the surgeons and their assistants make use of small manual retractors to pull muscles aside rather than cut them to allow better visualization of different parts of the field.

f. The surgeon uses the index finger of the nondominant hand to pull the thyroid lobe toward the midline (towards the trachea) and allowing visualization of vessels and structures lateral to the thyroid. At the same time as medial traction is placed on the thyroid, lateral retraction is placed on the strap muscles by the surgical assistant and carotid sheath allowing better visualization of the relationship of the inferior thyroidal vessels to the recurrent laryngeal nerve (RLN, the nerve to the voice box).

g. Once the lateral aspects of thyroid gland is exposed, the middle thyroid vein is identified and ligated, allowing the surgeon's non dominant hand to expose the inferior pole and superior poles of the thyroid.

h. The inferior pole of the thyroid is exposed revealing the inferior thyroidal artery and vein. The RLN can cross quite close to the posterior aspect of the inferior thyroidal vessels and the surgeon takes care to identify the RLN and avoid injury to it. The inferior thyroidal vessels are then ligated and disconnected directly at the level of the thyroid capsule. The surgeon is very careful to stay close to the thyroid capsule during the surgery thus protecting the RLN from injury and also allowing preservation of the vascular flow to the inferior parathyroids. As a general point this is a critical part of the operation because the important nerve to the voice box, the RLN usually crosses under the inferior thyroidal artery, but can occasionally travel over the artery, or in between the two branches of the inferior thyroid artery. The surgeon must know this anatomy including all the variations of the anatomy down pat.

i. The surgeon must be able to differentiate parathyroid from thyroid tissue. This can be somewhat challenging, though generally the parathyroids are enveloped in fat and are often a tan color. The inferior parathyroid can often be seen near the inferior pole vessels.

j. Further dissection allows further mobilization of the thyroid, and the superior pole vessels are also divided close to the capsule to avoid injury to the superior laryngeal nerve (SLN, a smaller nerve that controls more the pitch and projection of the voice.) The SLN also has a variety of patterns of travel prior to insertion into the cricothyroid muscle and the surgeon's knowledge of this anatomy is also important, especially if the patient uses their voice professionally or sings.

k. Once the superior and inferior pole vessels have been ligated, the thyroid gland is gently and carefully mobilized further now allowing further visualization of the structures posterior to the thyroid. Now the surgeon can see the ligament of Berry, the RLN, both parathyroids, and the narrow groove between the trachea and esophagus. During this part of the operation, delicate dissection is key to avoid tearing of any small branches of the inferior thyroid artery or undue pulling or pressure on the RLN. The ligament of Berry is a dense condensation of tissue including blood vessels that attaches the thyroid to the first and second tracheal rings. As a general rule, electric cautery is not used during this part of the dissection since cautery injury to the RLN is a real possibility. Small clips or fine silk ties can be used to divide these vessels. Care must be taken to stay tight to the thyroid gland. Sometimes thyroid tissue at this location may be found posteriorly behind the RLN, and the surgeon takes extreme care at this location not to injure the nerve. Sometimes, the surgeon feels it is safest to leave a small (1–2 mm) bit of thyroid behind rather than avoid injury to the RLN.

l. The final connections of the thyroid to the trachea are then divided and the thyroid isthmus (middle part) is divided using a surgical clamp and a silk suture ligature is used to control bleeding in the remaining one half of the thyroid. (See intraoperative photograph)

m. The surgeon inspects the removed half of the thyroid and marks it for the pathologist. The surgeon makes sure important information about the operative findings and the patient is communicated to the pathologist.

n. The surgeon checks the area for proper hemostasis, making sure there is no bleeding going on. At this point the trachea, RLN, cricothyroid muscle, SLN, and both parathyroids are exposed and must be treated very gently to avoid injury.

o. If the surgeon is using electric signals via a recurrent laryngeal nerve monitor to check integrity of the nerve one final check is made at this point.

p. If any of the parathyroids are thought to be dusky or ischemic, it can be removed by the surgeon then reimplanted into the large neck muscles.

q. Once hemostasis is verified, the strap muscle layers are reapproximated individually using suture. The more superficial platysma is closed similarly and the skin is closed using a plastic surgery technique where the sutures are not visible.

r. The surgeon applies a sterile dressing.

s. During emergence from anesthesia the surgeon is right at the bedside and is attentive to what is happening as the patient wakes up. Everyone is careful that the patient wakes up with no breathing or airway issue. Steps are taken to avoid retching during emergence from anesthesia since this can lead to bleeding.

6. The surgeon will be involved in the immediate postoperative management of the patient

a. The surgeon will make sure the head of the bed is elevated in the recovery room and that there is treatment of any postoperative nausea and vomiting. The surgeon and the nursing staff will make sure there are no issues with the airway or postoperative complications such as a neck hematoma. Some surgeons will measure serum calcium if a total thyroidectomy has been performed.

7. The surgeon will follow the patient and see the patient as an outpatient to discuss the final pathology and to look for any problems related to the surgery.

NOVEL HORIZONS IN THYROID SURGERY: MINIMALLY INVASIVE OR MAYBE NOT?

So far we have been talking about standards in thyroid surgery. Now we will talk about some approaches to thyroid surgery that are either fairly new or exceedingly new, in other words—cutting edge. Remember that traditional thyroidectomy is performed through a transverse cervical incision, and is associated with a very low morbidity and mortality rate. In other words, most patients do great. The one thing about thyroid surgery that still irks some patients and surgeons alike is having a scar on the neck. Though in most people the scar heals well, let's face it, having no scar would be even better. Not everyone is vain, especially when facing cancer, and most people just want the surgeon to do the best job possible, so the cancer has the lowest chance of recurring. However, the scar remaining after the procedure in such an exposed area as the neck is disliked by many patients, especially young women. During the 1990s, there was a surgical revolution and a general tendency to develop minimally invasive operations. Operations traditionally done with large incisions, such as gallbladder surgery and colon surgery, are now done routinely with an endoscopic approach using special camera equipment and small instruments put into the abdomen through small incisions. Often patients were pleased with the results since incisions were tiny, the recovery time was faster, and associated with significantly less pain. Naturally, endocrine surgeons were also part of this radical change in surgery and at first applied these minimally invasive techniques to *adrenalectomy* (removal of the adrenal glands which sit above the kidney) for certain adrenal tumors. Later, minimally invasive techniques were also tried for neck surgery including both parathyroidectomy and thyroidectomy. These techniques encompass a range of different minimally invasive surgical approaches. Sometimes a special camera (endoscope) is introduced through a smaller incision in the neck to allow better visualization and smaller instruments are used to take out the thyroid. Of all the minimally invasive approaches, this is the most wide spread, minimally invasive and is called a minimally invasive video-assisted thyroidectomy (MIVAT). It was set up, developed, and popularized by Dr. Paolo Miccoli's surgical team in Pisa, Italy (Miccoli, Berti et al. 2001). These procedures require some special instruments: an endoscope (30° or 45° angled rigid telescopes, 5 or 10 mm in diameter), endoscopic instruments, and trocars.

Remember that it is important that the outcome of the operation be no different whether the operation is done as a minimally invasive approach or through the traditional approach. The surgeon must get safe access to the thyroid, create a working space, dissect the thyroid lobe(s) after the identification of the recurrent nerve and the parathyroids, and then remove the thyroid lobe intact so

Personal Notes: Learning from Experience
Comments from a Thyroid Surgeon

Dr. Antonia Stephen is an instructor in surgery at Harvard Medical School and practices at the Massachusetts General Hospital in Boston. She is a sought-after endocrine surgeon and dedicates herself to meticulous care of patients who need surgery on the thyroid, parathyroid, or adrenal glands. She does research on use of ultrasound and fine needle aspiration in detecting thyroid cancers earlier. She lives in Boston with her husband and her three children. Here she writes a personal note about the trials and tribulations of becoming a thyroid surgeon and what keeps her going:

Thyroid surgery is an art and being a thyroid surgeon combines many aspects and talents. The pathway to becoming a thyroid surgeon includes four years of medical school, a surgical residency training program, and a fellowship focused on thyroid, parathyroid, and adrenal surgery. Although this may sound long and arduous, medical and surgical training is a fascinating adventure, filled with excitement, learning, and the formation of lifelong friendships. There is lots of hard work, of course, but the rewards are far greater. Once the training is completed, your days are spent seeing patients with thyroid problems, performing surgery, and often also working on research projects and other academic pursuits such as book chapters on thyroid surgery topics. Surgeons form a special bond with their patients and this bond begins with their initial or preoperative office visit. Often patients enter the office scared and nervous, and it is our role to reassure and at the same time educate and inform them about thyroid disease and thyroid surgery. We discuss with them everything from the technical aspects and possible risks, to when they can go back to work, drive a car, and lift their children after surgery. Being able to perform thyroid surgery itself is the most amazing aspect of being a thyroid surgeon. There are so many important structures in the neck, we must be careful not to injure any of them. For example, there are intricate nerves adjacent to the thyroid gland, including the primary ones innervating the vocal cords. If these nerves are cut, stretched, or in any other way damaged during the surgery, the patient may experience significant hoarseness. Fortunately, this does not happen very often, and one of the great challenges of this career path is locating those nerves and making sure they are kept intact. This keeps us on our toes every day.

Thyroid surgery is never boring. The best news about being a thyroid surgeon is that most thyroid conditions, even cancers, are curable, and it brings joy to us every day to see patients get well, get better, and live long and productive healthy lives, in part as a result of our work. There are very few emergencies, and once the residency training is completed, there is ample opportunity for a life outside the hospital, including being a hands-on Mom, which may be the only thing that is even harder, and more fun, than being a surgeon.

the pathologist can make a definitive diagnosis. In general, the vast majority of surgeons only perform traditional thyroidectomies, but the few who do use a minimally invasive approach, only do it for certain kinds of thyroid disease. Patients with small thyroid nodules that are under 2.5 cm (an inch or so) or a small multinodular goiter are reasonable candidates. Most surgeons still do not offer this procedure to patients with thyroid cancers as it is not clear whether surgeons can carefully separate the cancer from the nerve or check for any involved lymph nodes with the minimally invasive approach. Some diseases like thyroiditis or Graves' disease pose a relative contraindication to the minimally invasive approaches because of the inflammatory changes around the thyroid and a higher risk of intraoperative and postoperative bleeding. Patients with large or fat necks may also not be good candidates for these surgical approaches.

In addition to the MIVAT where the incision is smaller but still in the neck, two other main endoscopic approaches have been described for the thyroid gland: the axillary (Ikeda, Takami et al. 2000) and the breast approach (Choe, Kim et al. 2007). In the axillary approach, incisions are made in the armpit and an endoscope is guided up towards the thyroid gland in the neck where the surgery is done. This can be done with a standard endoscopic approach or sometimes with the help of a surgical robot. In the breast approach, small incisions are made just at the top of each nipple and the endoscope and other instruments are then tunneled up to the neck where a working space is created and the thyroid is removed. Many of these endoscopic approaches are done with the same instruments used for other abdominal surgeries, but some surgeons have used a surgical robot because of the ease of movement. Using a robot for surgery is a bit like playing a video game. The robot's surgical arms are placed into incisions made by the surgeon (for example, in the armpit area) and the surgeon then sits at a console that is far from the patient and uses special handles much like a video game to drive the robotic hands to do the actual surgery (Lee, Rao et al. 2009).

Other techniques have been described, such as the coming from behind the ear (Lee, Kim et al. 2009) or through the floor of the mouth (Benhidjeb, Wilhelm et al. 2009), but currently these are only in the experimental phase or performed in very limited number of patients and it is difficult to tell whether they are safe approaches or not.

What is surprising is that most of these minimally invasive surgery approaches are actually not all that minimally invasive. The surgery always requires general anesthesia, often takes a lot longer and is considerably more expensive. More importantly, in some cases the incisions, while placed in cosmetically appealing areas which hide scars well, such as the edge of the nipple or the armpit, necessitate that a long area along the chest wall be dissected which can be associated with higher rate of bleeding or infection. Furthermore, if there is a bleeding complication in the thyroid or anywhere in the track of the operation, then additional incisions may be needed (even in the neck) to control the bleeding. Bottom line is that most surgeons who perform thyroid surgery for a living, are a bit uncomfortable with all these potential complications when thyroid surgery done the traditional tried and tested way is so safe and really creates a pretty small neck incision. That having been said, surgeons are pretty innovative people especially when we think about how far our field has come, so a little navigation into unchartered waters may not be a terrible thing. Surgeons want to try new approaches to best serve their patients. Surgeon and patients must both always remember that the safety of the patient is the most important thing in all of this.

REFERENCES

Benhidjeb, T., T. Wilhelm, et al. (2009). "Natural orifice surgery on thyroid gland: totally transoral video-assisted thyroidectomy (TOVAT): report of first experimental results of a new surgical method." *Surg Endosc* **23**(5): 1119–20.

Choe, J. H., S. W. Kim, et al. (2007). "Endoscopic thyroidectomy using a new bilateral axillo-breast approach." *World J Surg* **31**(3): 601–6.

Halsted, W. (1920). "The operative story of goitre." *Johns Hopkins Hospital Report* **19**: 71.

Herr, H. W. (2007). "Ignorance is bliss: the Listerian revolution and education of American surgeons." J *Urol* **177**(2): 457–60.

Ikeda, Y., H. Takami, et al. (2000). "Endoscopic neck surgery by the axillary approach." J *Am Coll Surg* **191**(3): 336–40.

Lahey, F. H. and W. B. Hoover (1938). "Injuries to the recurrent laryngeal nerve in thyroid operations: their management and avoidance." *Ann Surg* **108**(4): 545–62.

Lee, K. E., H. Y. Kim, et al. (2009). "Postauricular and axillary approach endoscopic neck surgery: a new technique." *World J Surg* **33**(4): 767–72.

Lee, K. E., J. Rao, et al. (2009). "Endoscopic thyroidectomy with the da Vinci robot system using the bilateral axillary breast approach (BABA) technique: our initial experience." *Surg Laparosc Endosc Percutan Tech* **19**(3): e71–75.

McGreevy, P. S. and F. A. Miller (1969). "Biography of Theodor Kocher." *Surgery* **65**(6): 990–99.

Miccoli, P., P. Berti, et al. (2001). "Minimally invasive video-assisted thyroidectomy." *Am J Surg* **181**(6): 567–70.

Nobel Foundation. (2010). "Theodor Kocher, The Nobel Prize in Physiology or Medicine 1909," 2010, from http://nobelprize.org/nobel_prizes/medicine/laureates/1909/kocher-bio.html.

Shields, D. (1999). Historical landmarks in head and neck cancer surgery. American Head and Neck Society.

Spanknebel, K., J. A. Chabot, et al. (2005). "Thyroidectomy using local anesthesia: a report of 1,025 cases over 16 years." J *Am Coll Surg* **201**(3): 375–85.

Toledo, A. H. (2006). "John Collins Warren: master educator and pioneer surgeon of ether fame." *J Invest Surg* **19**(6): 341–44.

7

Long-Term Outlook

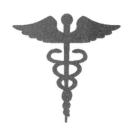

KEEPING YOUR THYROID HEALTHY: EVERY LITTLE BIT COUNTS

Most people don't really think of keeping their body parts healthy one at a time. Most of us just want to be healthy and live a long life free of diseases and with a minimum number of health issues. Some organs are more prone to damage just by virtue of where in the body they are located, such as your skin. Think of all the potential damaging things that happen to your skin every day, sunlight, radiation, extremes in temperature, salt, dangerous chemical exposures, etc. The truth is that most of our body parts have, through the millennia of evolution, developed a remarkable ability to protect themselves and stay healthy through thick and thin. There is however, some common sense things that we can all do to make sure our thyroids are functioning just right.

Many of the activities that keep your body healthy as a whole also serve to keep your thyroid healthy. Avoiding tobacco products, eating in moderation, regular exercise, and maintaining good sleep habits—all help to keep your thyroid in homeostatic balance. Avoiding obesity is one of the most important lifestyle goals for developing young adults. Extra adipose tissue (i.e., fat) increases the peripheral conversion of estrogen. Estrogen can stimulate thyroid nodule formation, which is one reason why thyroid disease is more common in woman compared to men.

The most important dietary recommendation to ensure a healthy thyroid is to eat iodine in moderate doses only. Most multivitamin preparations contain the recommended daily allowance of iodine, which is 100–150 mcg of iodine a day. A pregnant woman needs higher amounts (approximately 220–290 mcg of iodine/day) to help with fetal brain development. Many different types of food also contain iodine.

THE IMPORTANCE OF IODINE AND OTHER MINERALS TO THE THYROID GLAND: FEED THE NEED

Iodine is a naturally occurring chemical element that is an essential component of thyroid hormone. In the eighteenth century, iodine was harvested from seaweed or kelp. In modern times, there are only two primary sources of iodine. The first source is from a type of sedimentary rock called caliche. Caliche is a hardened deposit of calcium carbonate that also contains small amounts of sodium iodate and sodium iodide. The second source of modern iodine is from the brine (salt water) found in natural gas fields. It is important to mention that povidone iodine (commonly sold as Betadine in the pharmacy) products are sold as topical antiseptics to clean abrasions or wounds and are poisonous if eaten.

Certain plants are high in iodine due to their preference for environments that have high iodine content. These plants include seaweed, kelp, red kidney beans, lima beans, navy beans, pinto beans, cowpeas, horseradish, rhubarb, and potato skins (Miller 1998). Rice, grains, and cereals may have a high iodine content depending on soil conditions where it was grown. Certain foods that have additives from seaweed by-products include carrageenan, agar, alginate, and nori are also high in iodine. Other foodstuffs that are naturally high in iodine include egg yolks or any foods containing whole eggs (note: egg whites do not have very much iodine in them), red dye #3 (a common food additive), and blackstrap molasses (the product of the third boiling of molasses).

In addition, iodine is also used as a disinfectant against pathological bacteria in the dairy and bakery industry. Equipment in these production facilities is rinsed in a low concentration iodine solution prior to each use. Therefore, commercial large-scale bakery products and many dairy products including milk, powdered milk, cheese, cream, powdered dairy creamers, yogurt, butter, ice cream, whey, milk chocolate, and casein all contain small amounts of iodine (Pearce, Pino et al. 2004).

Certain types of foods block the absorption or utilization of iodine and should therefore also be eaten in moderation. These foods are called goiterogens because, if taken in very large amounts, they can cause a thyroid goiter to develop over time as the lack of iodine causes a drastic drop in thyroid hormone production. Soybeans and many different types of soy products including soymilk, soy sauce, and tofu can block iodine in high dosages. Interestingly, certain raw vegetables including turnips, cassava root, mustard greens, broccoli, cabbage, rutabaga, brussel sprouts, bok choy, cress, cauliflower, kale, and kohlrabi also inhibit iodine absorption. Cooking these vegetables deactivates the iodine blocking agents. It is widely believed that licorice root, which is used to flavor many different kinds of candy, may suppress thyroid function in large quantities. However, there are no articles in the medical literature to support this belief.

In addition to iodine, there are many other minerals and trace elements that are important to maintaining a healthy thyroid. For example, cobalt is a relatively rare magnetic element that is found in trace amounts in fish, nuts, cereals, and green leafy vegetables. Cobalt is also a major component of vitamin B12 so the recommended daily allowance of cobalt for an adult is the same as the normal amount of B12 for an adult (1.5 mcg/day). Excessive amounts of cobalt may produce goiter and reduce thyroid activity (Barceloux 1999).

Certain natural elements are needed to prevent thyroid disease. These elements include copper, manganese, boron, zinc, magnesium, bromine, and iron (Allain, Berre et al. 1993). There is a large amount of evidence in the medical literature that iron deficiency reduces thyroid hormone synthesis by decreasing the activity of thyroid peroxidase, and that iron supplementation improves the efficacy of iodine supplementation (Zimmermann and Kohrle 2002). On the other hand, heavy metals such as cadmium, lead, chromium, and mercury (found in old dental amalgams) may predispose to thyroid disease for unclear reasons.

There has also been a great deal of medical research into the trace element selenium. Selenium is an essential trace element that is found in wheat germ, seafood and shellfish, beef liver and kidney, eggs, sunflower and sesame seeds, Brazil nuts, mushrooms, garlic, onions, and kelp. Selenium is used for cellular anti-oxidative defense systems and may function to protect the thyroid gland from attack by excess hydrogen peroxide and reactive oxygen molecules generated during the production of thyroid hormone. Selenium is also a key portion of the deiodinases that are used to convert T4 to T3. Therefore it is not surprising that the thyroid gland has the one of the highest selenium content per mass unit of any organ in the human body. Fortunately, it is difficult to have selenium deficiency unless an individual is receiving total parenteral nutrition (liquid nutrition through the veins) or in certain chronic disease states with decreased gastrointestinal absorption of selenium such as cystic fibrosis or phenylketouria (Kohrle and Gartner 2009).

One More Thing to Know: Now That's Interesting
The Wolff-Chaikoff Effect:
Thyroid Protector in the Event of Nuclear Catastrophe

In 1948, Drs. Jan Wolff and Israel Lyon Chaikoff in the division of physiology at the University of California at Berkley published their observations on the effect of blood iodine levels on the regulation of thyroid function in rats (Wolff and Chaikoff 1948). They noted that raising the level of iodine in the blood above a critical level, results in almost complete blockage of organic binding of iodine within the rat's thyroid gland. This result was coined the "Wolff-Chaikoff Effect," but had actually been published by Dr. Chaikoff's laboratory several years earlier in 1944 with slices of sheep thyroid glands (Morton, Chaikoff et al. 1944). However, their 1948 study was the first proof of the negative effect of excess iodine on the thyroid function of a living animal. The next year, Dr. Chaikoff's laboratory published a follow-up study that described how the Wolff-Chaikoff effect appeared to only last 26–50 hours in rats despite high blood concentrations of iodine (Wolff, Chaikoff et al. 1949). The temporary nature of the Wolff-Chaikoff effect, despite high levels of iodine, was termed an "escape phenomenon."

Now, over 60 years later, the Wolff-Chaikoff effect is still believed to be an important feature of the human auto-regulation of thyroid hormone production during periods of exposure to high levels of iodine. Large amounts of intra-thyroidal iodine inhibit iodine transport, hydrogen peroxide generation, iodide organification, and thyroid hormone secretion through molecular regulatory mechanisms that are not clear, but may be due to special forms of iodine-saturated fatty acids that are formed within the thyroid called iodolipids (Dugrillon 1996).

The most direct application of the Wolff-Chaikoff effect for humans would be in the event of a nuclear accident or war. Radiation exposure to the thyroid can lead to the development of thyroid cancer (see Chapter 5 on thyroid cancer). Therefore, in the event of a nuclear accident or war, large amounts of potassium iodine would be distributed to any survivors to induce the Wolff-Chaikoff effect. In the 1960s, at the height of the Cold War between the United States and the former Soviet Union, numerous fallout shelters were constructed underneath homes and schools across the world and stocked with numerous supplies of potassium iodide pills. Taking potassium iodide shortly after radiation exposure would essentially shut down all thyroid activity and protect the thyroid from any absorbed radiation. The escape phenomenon would allow thyroid activity to resume several days later, presumably after the survivors have been removed from the source of radiation exposure or radiation levels had decreased (Zanzonico and Becker 2000).

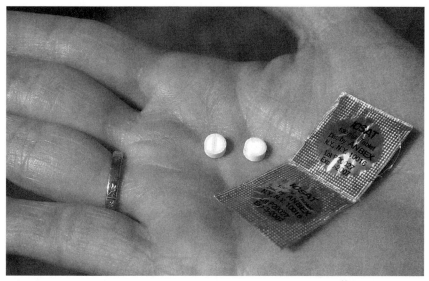

Potassium iodide pills taken immediately after an accidental radiation exposure can help protect the thyroid and reduce the chance of thyroid cancer. (AP Photo/Carlos T. Miranda)

IMPACT OF OTHER MEDICATIONS ON THE HEALTH OF THE THYROID: ANOTHER EXAMPLE OF POLYPHARMACY

Some types of medications and herbal supplements may affect overall thyroid function. Anti-depressants are commonly prescribed and many affect thyroid function. Selective serotonin reuptake inhibitors (SSRIs) such as fluoxetine (Prozac), sertraline (Zoloft), citalopram (Celexa), and paroxetine (Paxil) are used for the treatment of clinical depression. However, long-term use of SSRIs may cause an elevation in TSH levels with subsequent overstimulation of the thyroid gland and eventual decrease in overall thyroid hormone levels (Gitlin, Altshuler et al. 2004). Tricyclic antidepressants (TCAs) are also used in the treatment of depression and may negatively affect thyroid function. TCAs such as amitriptyline (Elavil), nortriptyline (Pamelor), and Clomipramine (Anafranil) interfere with normal thyroid function by binding to iodine and preventing it from being used for thyroid hormone synthesis, directly decreasing thyroid peroxidase activity, or by enhancing the deiodination of T4 to T3 by stimulating deiodinase activity (Sauvage, Marquet et al. 1998). The medications lithium and amiodorone have already been discussed in Chapter 3. Finally, certain anti-epileptic medications including cabamazepine, oxcarbazepine, phenytoin, and barbiturates may reduce serum levels of T3 or T4. Interestingly, this reduction in serum thyroid hormone levels does not appear to result in clinical hypothyroidism even with long-term use for unclear reasons (Steinhoff 2006).

Finally, herbal supplements such as ginseng and St. John's wort (*hypericum perforatum*) may cause an elevation in thyroid stimulating hormone levels with subsequent overstimulation of the thyroid gland with long-term use (Ferko and Levine 2001). More research is needed to determine the mechanism for this possible effect on thyroid function.

THYROID DISEASE AND PREGNANCY: AN INTRICATE BALANCE

During pregnancy there is a natural fluctuation in hormones that can change the overall function of the thyroid gland. *Human chorionic gonadotropin (hCG)* and estrogen levels are greatly increased during pregnancy and both can stimulate the thyroid gland to produce more thyroid hormone and therefore decrease the amounts of TSH in the blood. More thyroid hormone is needed during pregnancy, as the baby is completely dependent on the mother's thyroid hormone levels until at least the 12th week of gestation. The increase in thyroid function can also cause the thyroid to swell in size slightly during pregnancy (10–15% bigger on average) that should resolve once the baby is delivered. As mentioned previously in this chapter, it is important for women to consume at least 200 mcg of iodine a day (twice the normal daily amount) during pregnancy to keep up with this increase in thyroid activity.

Interestingly, pregnancies can sometimes "unmask" or reveal subclinical thyroid disease that was already present in the mother. This is especially true for women who may have had subclinical hypothyroidism from Hashimoto's Disease prior to the pregnancy. In other words, a woman may have had barely enough thyroid hormone for herself before she was pregnant, and now that she is pregnant, her thyroid cannot make enough thyroid hormone for both her and the baby. Severe hypothyroidism during pregnancy can have serious complications for both the mom and the baby including increasing the risk of miscarriage, bleeding, muscle weakness, congestive heart failure, and visual-motor or intelligence deficiencies in the developing baby.

Alternatively, women who had subclinical hyperthyroid disease may also experience a worsening of symptoms due to the increased thyroid stimulation during pregnancy. This phenomenon is especially common in women with Graves' disease. Untreated severe hyperthyroidism during pregnancy can lead to early labor, *pre-eclampsia* (a serious combination of fluid retention and hypertension that can lead to eclampsia, which is characterized by seizures and coma), and thyroid storm. Hyperthyroidism during pregnancy due to Graves' disease can also have serious consequences for the baby including complete suppression of the baby's thyroid formation and function, low birth weight, and prematurity.

Unfortunately, the various hormonal fluctuations that occur with pregnancy can make the interpretation of thyroid function testing more difficult than normal. Therefore, there is still no general consensus among various medical organizations about the cost-effectiveness of screening all pregnant women. Some groups only recommend screening for women at high risk for developing thyroid disease (known thyroid disease before pregnancy, history of radiation exposure to the neck, presence of autoimmune diseases, family history of thyroid disease, and presence of a goiter) (Abalovich, Amino et al. 2007; Schroeder 2002). Other groups have recommended universal screening of pregnant women preferably during the first trimester (Gharib, Tuttle et al. 2005). A recent randomized, prospective study in Italy compared universal screening versus only screening in women for high risk of thyroid disease in 4,562 women and found no difference in adverse outcomes by screening all women (Negro, Schwartz et al. 2010). Further large, multicenter trials will be required before this issue can be laid to rest.

In summary, many of the activities that serve to keep your body happy and healthy also help to keep your thyroid gland happy and healthy. These activities include exercise, maintaining an appropriate diet, avoiding polypharmacy, and receiving pre-natal care while pregnant.

REFERENCES

Abalovich, M., N. Amino, et al. (2007). "Management of thyroid dysfunction during pregnancy and postpartum: an Endocrine Society Clinical Practice Guideline." *J Clin Endocrinol Metab* **92**(8 Suppl): S1–47.

Allain, P., S. Berre, et al. (1993). "Bromine and thyroid hormone activity." *J Clin Pathol* **46**(5): 456–58.

Barceloux, D. G. (1999). "Cobalt." *J Toxicol Clin Toxicol* **37**(2): 201–6.

Dugrillon, A. (1996). "Iodolactones and iodoaldehydes—mediators of iodine in thyroid autoregulation." *Exp Clin Endocrinol Diabetes* **104** (Suppl 4): 41–45.

Ferko, N. and M. A. Levine (2001). "Evaluation of the association between St. John's wort and elevated thyroid-stimulating hormone." *Pharmacotherapy* **21**(12): 1574–78.

Gharib, H., R. M. Tuttle, et al. (2005). "Consensus Statement #1: Subclinical thyroid dysfunction: a joint statement on management from the American Association of Clinical Endocrinologists, the American Thyroid Association, and The Endocrine Society." *Thyroid* **15**(1): 24–28; response 32–33.

Gitlin, M., L. L. Altshuler, et al. (2004). "Peripheral thyroid hormones and response to selective serotonin reuptake inhibitors." *J Psychiatry Neurosci* **29**(5): 383–86.

Kohrle, J. and R. Gartner (2009). "Selenium and thyroid." *Best Pract Res Clin Endocrinol Metab* **23**(6): 815–27.

Miller, L. G. (1998). "Herbal medicinals: selected clinical considerations focusing on known or potential drug-herb interactions." *Arch Intern Med* **158**(20): 2200–11.

Morton, M. E., I. L. Chaikoff, et al. (1944). "Inhibiting effect of inorganic iodide on the formation of in vitro thyroxine and diiodotyrosine by surviving thyroid tissue." *J Biol Chem* **164**(2): 381–87.

Negro, R., A. Schwartz, et al. (Apr 2010). "Universal screening versus case finding for detection and treatment of thyroid hormonal dysfunction during pregnancy." *J Clin Endocrinol Metab* **95**(4): 1699–707.

Pearce, E. N., S. Pino, et al. (2004). "Sources of dietary iodine: bread, cows' milk, and infant formula in the Boston area." *J Clin Endocrinol Metab* **89**(7): 3421–24.

Sauvage, M. F., P. Marquet, et al. (1998). "Relationship between psychotropic drugs and thyroid function: a review." *Toxicol Appl Pharmacol* **149**(2): 127–35.

Schroeder, B. M. (2002). "ACOG practice bulletin on thyroid disease in pregnancy." *Am Fam Physician* **65**(10): 2158, 2161–62.

Steinhoff, B. J. (2006). "Optimizing therapy of seizures in patients with endocrine disorders." *Neurology* **67**(12 Suppl 4): S23–27.

Wolff, J. and I. L. Chaikoff (1948). "Plasma inorganic iodide, a chemical regulator of normal thyroid function." *Endocrinology* **42**(6): 468–71.

Wolff, J., I. L. Chaikoff, et al. (1949). "The temporary nature of the inhibitory action of excess iodine on organic iodine synthesis in the normal thyroid." *Endocrinology* **45**(5): 504–13, illust.

Zanzonico, P. B. and D. V. Becker (2000). "Effects of time of administration and dietary iodine levels on potassium iodide (KI) blockade of thyroid irradiation by 131I from radioactive fallout." *Health Phys* **78**(6): 660–67.

Zimmermann, M. B. and J. Kohrle (2002). "The impact of iron and selenium deficiencies on iodine and thyroid metabolism: biochemistry and relevance to public health." *Thyroid* **12**(10): 867–78.

8

Current Research on the Thyroid

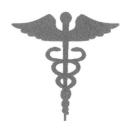

CURRENT RESEARCH IN THYROID CANCER: LEAVE NO STONE UNTURNED

Medical researchers often choose projects that interest them for their research and certainly researchers working on the thyroid gland have had their share of important medical discoveries in the past 100 years. Much of what is understood about the thyroid gland came through the hard work of all kinds of medical researchers and physicians; many of these contributions were highlighted in the chapters dealing with the physiology, anatomy, and surgery of the thyroid gland. In this chapter, we will focus on the most up-to date-research in thyroid diseases and give small samples of some of them most exciting ones.

Thyroid cancer research runs the gamut from genetic predispositions, early diagnosis, new more sensitive imaging tools, how to make the diagnosis more accurately, to safer surgical procedures and post-operative targeted treatments. As in other cancers, the role of certain abnormal genes and proteins in leading normal cells in the thyroid to become cancerous and go into overdrive with the ability to metastasize and travel to other organs, is an intense subject of investigation. When thyroid cells transform to a malignant state, lots of changes are seen in the genes of the cells and some of these quite specific to a particular kind of thyroid cancer. These changes are called *mutations* and common pathways of altered genes for the two most common forms of thyroid cancer are shown in Figure 8.1. Most of these mutations give the thyroid cell some kind of advantage, leading it to over-grow its bounds and sometimes the mutations can lead the cell to develop brand new capabilities that can really cause havoc in the thyroid and neighboring healthy tissues. Normally thyroid cells know to stay inside the thyroid and have a low rate of growth (cellular division), but sometimes even small genetic changes can lead to a chain of events which can lead to catastrophic results. For example, a one unit change in even a single gene nucleotide (the smallest building block of the cell's DNA) can lead to a major change in proteins produced in the cell such that thyroid cells suddenly start making enzymes that cause the cells to eat through the lining of the thyroid and into adjacent blood vessels to gain access to the vascular system. These cells then travel in the blood, something they other-wise would never do, and settle into other areas of the body such as lung tissue and bones. These new deposits of thyroid cells are called metastases, and once they take hold and grow, they can destroy the organ where they have settled in; the bot-tom line is that thyroid cells belong only in the thyroid and should not be growing anywhere else. The initiating events in this complex series of cellular changes as well as every one of the following steps are the subject of intense study. In the fol-lowing sections, we will discuss the genetic changes that can mislead a normal thy-roid cell down the path to becoming a destructive cancerous cell. There is a lot more research in thyroid diseases and thyroid cancer, but our discussion will focus on the genetic changes in each of the thyroid tumors we have studied in earlier chapters.

CURRENT RESEARCH IN PAPILLARY THYROID CANCER

Important discoveries about the molecular origins of papillary thyroid cancer have been made in the last decade. Specifically, we now realize that most papil-lary thyroid cancers are due to activating mutations in one of three possible genes: BRAF, RAS, and RET/PTC rearrangements (see Figure 8.1). Let's look at each of these genes closely.

The BRAF gene normally makes a protein called B-RAF, which is shorthand scientific notation for V-raf murine sarcoma viral oncogene homolog B1. This protein is a kinase that closely regulates cellular growth and division through the MAPK pathway (mitogen-activated protein kinases). An activating muta-tion in the BRAF gene at position 1796 may lead to excess BRAF protein pro-duction and therefore uncontrolled cellular growth. Also, BRAF mutation may lead to a loss of the thyrocyte's ability to import iodide molecules (Durante,

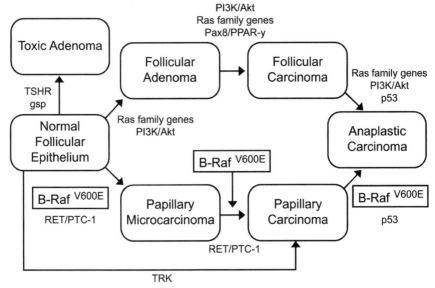

Figure 8.1   Common genetic mutations seen during the progression of a variety of different thyroid cancers. (Drawn by Jeff Dixon after Dr. Sareh Parangi, MD)

Puxeddu et al. 2007), which is a possible explanation for why many aggressive thyroid cancers become refractory to radioactive iodine treatment (Xing, Westra et al. 2005).

The RAS gene stands for RAt Sarcoma gene and codes for more than a hundred different proteins that control intracellular signaling. An activating mutation of RAS genes may lead to increased invasion or metastasis of thyroid cancer cells into surrounding tissues and organs. Also, an activating RAS mutation may prevent thyroid cancer cells from undergoing normal cellular apoptosis or cell death. This process creates thyroid cancer cells that are "immortal" and continue growing until they surpass their blood and nutrient supplies.

Finally, activating mutations in the *proto-oncogene* called "rearranged during transfection" or RET for short, may lead to both papillary and medullary thyroid cancer. A proto-oncogene is a normal gene that when mutated becomes an *oncogene* (cancer-causing gene), which can subsequently convert a healthy cell into a cancer cell. Proto-oncogenes typically help cells to create proteins that are used to guide cellular growth and differentiation. If the proto-oncogene becomes mutated and begins to release too much of these proteins, cellular growth can be uncontrolled, which may lead to the development of a cancerous tumor. More about this process will be discussed later in the medullary thyroid cancer section.

CURRENT RESEARCH IN FOLLICULAR THYROID CANCER

PAX8 stands for paired box gene 8 and codes for a protein that is specifically involved in thyroid follicular cell development. Interestingly, mutations in PAX8 can cause it to become fused with PPAR-gamma (peroxisome proliferator-activated receptor gamma), which is a receptor protein that normally regulates glucose metabolism. The fusion of PAX8/PPAR-gamma is believed to stimulate cell division and eventually lead to the development of follicular carcinoma. Interestingly, the fusion of PAX8/PPAR-gamma has been found in up to 50 percent of follicular carcinomas, but not in follicular adenomas or papillary thyroid cancers (Lui, Foukakis et al. 2005). Future research may find an efficient method to test fine-needle aspiration biopsy specimens for follicular carcinoma, which would avoid removal of benign follicular adenomas. A preoperative diagnosis of follicular carcinoma would also allow a planned total thyroidectomy on initial operation and avoid the current need for completion thyroidectomy when a follicular carcinoma is diagnosed on final pathology.

CURRENT RESEARCH IN MEDULLARY THYROID CANCER

There have been several recent advances regarding the molecular origins of medullary thyroid cancer. As mentioned in Chapter 5, in 25 percent of cases, medullary thyroid cancer is associated with multiple endocrine neoplasia or familial medullary thyroid carcinoma. In the case of medullary thyroid cancer, the RET proto-oncogene mutation causes a special cellular receptor called a tyrosine kinase receptor to be constantly activated. Tyrosine is an amino acid that is one of the building blocks used by cells to create proteins. Kinases are special enzymes that are in charge of phosphorylation, which is the transfer of phosphate groups from high-energy molecules such as adenosine triphosphate (ATP) to substrate or target molecules. A *tyrosine kinase receptor* is a protein on a cell's surface that when activated causes the phosphorylation of tyrosine into proteins that stimulate cellular growth. Therefore, a mutation that causes a tyrosine kinase mutation to always be on eventually leads to a variety of cancers including medullary thyroid cancer.

NEW AGENTS FOR THE TREATMENT OF MEDULLARY CANCER: THE PROMISE OF TARGETED THERAPIES

As mentioned in Chapter 5, metastatic medullary thyroid cancer is resistant to traditional radiation and chemotherapies. Therefore, new therapies have been devised based on the most up to date knowledge about the genetics of medullary cancer. The specific gene rearrangements and protein structure alterations that result from them have lead to development of new therapies called *targeted therapies*. These targeted therapies target specific changed proteins and do not just try to kill growing cells like more traditional agents such as chemotherapy and radiation. A new treatment against metastatic medullary thyroid cancer is the use of tyrosine kinase inhibitors, which specifically block the activation effect of RET proto-oncogene mutations on tyrosine kinase receptors. Vandetanib, sorafenib, sunitinib, motesanib, and XL184 have shown the earliest promise. Based upon it's inhibitory activity against RET, as well as Vascular Endothelial Growth Factor (VEGF) and Epidermal Growth Factor Receptor (EGFR), vandetanib was studied in hereditary medullary thyroid cancer with preliminary data indicating good rates of objective response and disease stabilization (Wells and Santoro 2009). The promise of these agents in early studies has led to an international placebo-controlled phase III study (tests an experimental medication against a pill that looks like the medication, but does not have any active ingredients) in more than 200 patients with sporadic or hereditary advanced MTC. Although the results of large, randomized-controlled multi-institutional trials are not available at the time of publication of this book, preliminary studies indicate that tyrosine kinase inhibitors, such as motesanib, may be a safe method to prevent the growth of metastatic hereditary medullary thyroid cancers (Schlumberger, Elisei et al. 2009). Reports of small numbers of MTC patients responding to other VEFGR TKIs, such as sorafenib, sunitinib, axitinib, and XL184 confirm that this class of agents has clear activity in medullary thyroid cancer. Of these, XL184, which inhibits VEGFR2, C-MET, and RET, showed particular promise in an early study.

CURRENT RESEARCH IN ANAPLASTIC THYROID CANCER

Recently, there have been numerous discoveries regarding the molecular pathogenesis of anaplastic thyroid cancer. Although anaplastic thyroid cancer may develop *de novo* (Latin for "from the beginning"), it appears that the majority of anaplastic thyroid cancers arise from pre-existing well-differentiated thyroid cancers. The process of dedifferentiation from a well-differentiated thyroid cancer to an anaplastic thyroid cancer is likely due to the accumulation of genetic mutations. Early mutations include RAS and BRAF mutations as described earlier in this chapter for papillary thyroid cancer. Late mutations include the TP53 tumor suppressor gene, catenin, and PIK3CA. Let's look at each of these mutations more closely.

The TP53 tumor suppressor gene is located on the 17th human chromosome and normally is a cell cycle regulator. It gets its name from the fact that it is a tumor protein that is 53 kilodaltons in size. When human cells grow, they eventually reach a size where cellular reproduction is possible. TP53 is the police

---

One More Thing to Know:
Families with Medullary Cancer Saved from Early Death—How Mutation Testing
Lead to Prevention of Medullary Thyroid Cancer

Ever since James Watson and Francis Crick's work led to the discovery of DNA, scientists have worked furiously to use information contained in the DNA of every person to help with diseases. There are actually very few diseases though where genetic information has been transformed to an actual cure or even prevention of near certain death from disease. Here is a story which tells about one such discovery where eventually genetic changes in individuals is used to predict who will develop medullary cancer, a lethal form of thyroid cancer, if not detected very early in its course.

In 1956, Drs. Joe Tjio and Albert Levan accidentally discovered that the addition of a drop of water to human mitotic cells allowed the chromosomes to spread apart into easily counted separate forms (Tjio 1956). This fortuitous discovery enabled these two researchers to determine that the human genome has 46 chromosomes and establish the new field of human cytogenetics. Since then, technologies such as flow cytometry, biochemical fluorescence, and chromosomal arrays allow small mutations to be located across the entire human genome (Trask 2002). Some of these mutations can cause lethal diseases later in life, so it would be important to detect these diseases as early as possible if a cure was available.

In 1993, researchers determined that the genetic cause for hereditary medullary thyroid cancer were activating mutations in the Rearranged during Transfection proto-oncogene. Patients with Multiple Endocrine Neoplasia Type 2 (MEN-2-medullary thyroid cancer, pheochromocytoma, and primary hyperparathyroidism) have a nearly 100 percent chance of developing medullary thyroid cancer at some point in their lifetime. Unfortunately, prior to the development of genetic testing, patients would often present in adulthood with metastatic medullary thyroid cancer that was incurable because it had spread too far to be surgically removed. The development of a genetic screening tool now allows for the very early diagnosis of hereditary medullary thyroid cancer in children at high risk for carrying the MEN2 mutations. If these tests are positive, surgeons can then prophylactically remove the child's thyroid gland *before* the thyroid cancer has had a chance to develop. Therefore, thanks to genetic testing, a once lethal disease of adults has been converted into a curable procedure that is done in childhood (Sanso, Domene et al. 2002; Danko and Skinner 2006; Szinnai, Sarnacki et al. 2007).

---

officer of the cellular world and prevents uncontrolled cellular reproduction. Without TP53 cells, we would eventually accumulate too many mutations that would ultimately form into cancers. The protective role of the TP53 gene is why it is sometimes called the "guardian of the genome" or "master watchman"

(Read and Strachan 1999). Mutations in the TP53 gene are inactivating which subsequently allows cancers such as anaplastic thyroid cancer to form. TP53 gene mutations have been found in as many as 55 percent of all anaplastic thyroid cancers (Nikiforov 2004).

Catenin is a protein that plays a vital role in cellular adhesion. If cells were like Lego plastic blocks, catenin would be the small bumps on the top of the blocks that allow each block to attach to another block. Mutations in catenin cause a loss in the ability of one cell to adhere to another cell. If the cell was already a cancer cell from other mutations, then a loss of cellular adhesion would allow the cancer cell to spread to other parts of the body via the bloodstream or through the lymphatic system. Recent research has demonstrated that mutations in catenin may be present in up to 82 percent of anaplastic thyroid cancers (Kurihara, Ikeda et al. 2004).

PIK3CA is a human oncogene that creates a protein that is a portion of a larger enzymatic protein called phosphatidylinositol 3-kinase (PI3K for short). PI3Ks interact with insulin receptors to help regulate glucose uptake and cellular growth and survival. The details of this process are not entirely clear, but gain-in-function mutations in PIK3CA have been found in up to 63 percent of anaplastic thyroid cancers (Liu, Hou et al. 2008).

Unfortunately, the survival of people with anaplastic thyroid cancer has not changed dramatically despite increasing knowledge of the molecular pathogenesis and more aggressive chemo- and radiotherapies. In the future, the treatment of anaplastic thyroid cancer will likely require individualized treatment regimens after comprehensive tumor genetic testing. These treatment regimens will likely involve chemotherapies that feature drug delivery systems that are able to deliver very high concentrations of anti-cancer medications while minimizing toxic systemic side effects.

BASIC LABORATORY RESEARCH IN THYROID CANCER: FROM BENCH TO BEDSIDE

Much of what scientists have learned in the last few decades about the behavior of thyroid cancer has been by studying each and every step required to transform a normal thyroid cell into a cancerous cells. Cancer is a complex collection of diseases that feature unregulated or uncontrolled cellular growth. Normal body cells have a well-regulated system of cellular growth, cellular division, and then eventually cellular death. Adult cells typically reproduce only to replace worn-out or injured cells. On the other hand, cancer cells become "immortal" in the sense that they ignore normal cellular growth controls and continue to grow and divide even at the expense of surrounding cells. Non-blood cancer cells cluster together and eventually form a detectable lump once there are at least a billion cancer cells. Cancer cells may also acquire the ability to travel to other parts of the body and forming new colonies of cancer cells. This process of moving to other parts of the body is called *metastasis*, which is a derivation of the Greek word "methistanai," which means, "to change."

Some seemingly simple questions that naturally come to mind when dealing with cancer cells are actually incredibly complex when studied in the laboratory. For example, patient with thyroid cancer may ask themselves or their doctor some of these very logical questions:

- How come my normal thyroid cells started growing so fast?
- Why don't thyroid cancer cells just grow so fast that they burn themselves out?
- How do thyroid cells escape the out of my thyroid and travel in my blood-stream and metastasize to my lungs?
- How could thyroid cells actually survive in the lung? Don't they know where they belong?
- Why doesn't my immune system destroy cancer cells?

Many of these steps have been dissected in the laboratory using painstaking difficult techniques. Scientist studying thyroid cancer might focus on only these steps for decades. Some researchers work on how the cancer cells can be kept in check and contained inside the thyroid by normal surrounding thyroid tissue; while others work on reversing some of the genetic or enzymatic changes that occur inside the cancer cells; and yet others work on general mechanisms of cancer suppression such as strengthening the person's immune system to kill off the cancer cells as soon as they start traveling in the bloodstream. In order to understand the difficult job of studying these events, let's look at some of these steps more carefully.

First let's look at metastasis, whereby cancer cells grow out of the thyroid and move to a distant site such as bone or lung. This single action of a few or a few hundred cells leaving their organ of origin (i.e., the thyroid in this case) is actually very complex: the cancerous cells actually undertake a complex series of steps in which cancer cells leave the original tumor site and migrate to other parts of the body via the bloodstream or the lymphatic system. First the cells have to eat out of their usual home (the thyroid); then they actually have to make it into the bloodstream and survive. Later they have to figure out where they need to come back out of the bloodstream such as inside another body part like lung or bone, and then they have to travel back across the blood vessel in the new organ such as lung, settling into the new secondary location. In this new location, the thyroid cancer cells now need to recruit new blood vessels, acclimate themselves, and start growing again. It has taken scientist many years of hard work and hundreds of millions of dollars to slowly analyze each of these steps for some common cancers.

To initiate the first of these steps, malignant cells develop special enzymatic powers that allow them to break away from the primary tumor and attach to and degrade certain protein barriers that make up the surrounding extracellular matrix (ECM), which separates the tumor from adjoining normal tissue. By breaking down and degrading these proteins, cancer cells are able to breach the thyroid capsule and escape. When thyroid cancers metastasize, they commonly travel through the lymph system to the lymph nodes in the neck or directly into a blood vessel where they can get carried away to other parts of the body such as the lung, bone, or brain. The body can also resists metastasis by a variety of mechanisms through the actions of a class of proteins known as suppressors of tumor metastasis.

Cancer researchers studying the conditions necessary for cancer metastasis have discovered that one of the critical events required is the growth of a new network of blood vessels, called tumor *angiogenesis or lymphangiogenesis* (Folkman 1992). It has been found that natural products that are abundant in the normal thyroid tissue called *angiogenesis inhibitors* can normally therefore prevent the growth of metastases (Folkman 1996).

Angiogenesis, the formation of new blood vessels from existing vessels, is important in many benign and malignant diseases (Iruela-Arispe and Dvorak 1997). It is therefore no surprise that the process of angiogenesis in the thyroid gland is proving to be an important regulator of both benign and malignant thyroid conditions. In adults, new blood vessels are produced only through angiogenesis since the adult vasculature is normally quiescent except for highly ordered processes such as ovulation, implantation of the fertilized egg, pregnancy, and wound healing. The balance between stimulators and inhibitors of angiogenesis is a tightly regulated process that allows for no angiogenesis in normal adult tissues. Once this balance is disturbed, either through an increase in stimulatory signals or a decrease in inhibitory signals, then angiogenesis will begin. Stimulators of angiogenesis are special factors often produced by the cancer cells themselves that turn on angiogenesis and cause active recruitment of new blood vessels. These stimulators are potent chemical signal that start the growth of new blood vessels where there should be none. The process of angiogenesis is highly complex and involves signals from the surrounding matrix, stroma, epithelial tissue, as well as the *endothelial cell* (the cell lining the blood vessel) itself. This process is becoming more thoroughly understood and is clearly a complex physiologic process. The new blood vessel cells must coordinate not only cytoskeletal changes required for motility (movement of the cell) but also secretion of proteolytic enzymes to promote matrix degradation and invasion. We can simplify the steps of angiogenesis or how thyroid tumor cells manage to call for and get more blood vessels down to these basic steps:

- Thyroid cancer cells send out a special chemical signal to nearby blood vessels, this is a signal that stimulates angiogenesis, also known as a *proangiogenic* signal.
- Initial degradation of the basement membrane of the pre-existing nearby vessels.
- Sprouting of new vessel buds from the nearby vessels—kind of like buds on a tree.
- Sudden growth spurt of the endothelial cells—endothelial proliferation.
- Migration of the newly formed blood vessels cells towards the cancer cells—the new cells essentially start marching towards the source of the special chemical.
- New tube formation, the new blood vessel cells must coordinate not only cytoskeletal changes required for motility and additional cellular signals allowing for anchorage and formation of small tubes from the new invading endothelial cells.

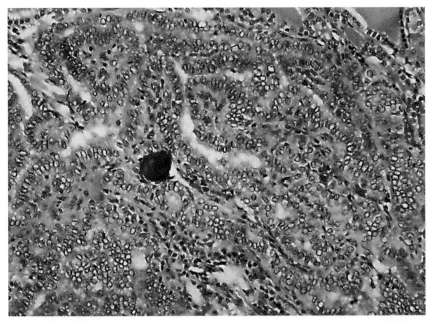

Papillary thyroid cancer has a fairly classic appearance under the microscope. (CDC/ Dr. Edwin P. Ewing, Jr.)

- Stabilization of the new vessel's basement membrane which can then provide signals to help maintain the new endothelium. The newly formed vessel then becomes responsive to its surrounding environment. The final size and density of the newly formed microvasculature is regulated by the genetic programming in the surrounding tissue, but is also fine tuned to the physiologic needs of the cancer cells that recruited the new blood vessels.

During tumor angiogenesis, the coordinated effort between growth factors, adhesion molecules, extracellular matrix proteins, and proteases lacks the organization that is found in normal physiologic angiogenesis such as is found in pregnancy. The resultant vessels lack coordinated regulation and can be poorly organized but still play an essential role in allowing the tumor to grow big.

Researchers are spending a great deal of energy attempting to discern which exact proangiogenic factors are involved in the pathogenesis of various thyroid malignancies, how these differences may be responsible for their unique clinical characteristics, and how this knowledge can be utilized to develop new therapies.

The formation of new lymphatic vessels is very similar to that of new blood vessel formation but the two networks are both functionally and structurally distinct. Blood vessels function in delivery of nutrients, oxygen and immune cells, whereas the lymphatics take up interstitial fluid that gets left over in the tissue containing immune cells and spilled proteins and filter them through lymph nodes eventually returning them to the circulatory system. Structurally, lymphatics are larger than blood vessels, are thinner walled. A lot of researchers have always focused on blood vessels, but more recently there is a surge of research on how tumors might recruit lymphatic channels in order to spread. It seems tumors can lead to *lymphangiogenesis* thereby promoting metastasis, such as tumor formation. Studies looking at the role tumor cells have in initiating angiogenesis versus lymphangiogenesis has been hampered by the limitations in our ability to accurately distinguish lymphatics from blood vessel endothelium, especially in the setting of a tumor. In other words, we don't have very good special markers or stains that can tell lymphatics from blood vessels. *Chemokine* receptor signaling is one potential mechanism by which a tumor cell interacts with the lymphatic endothelium in order to metastasize into the lymphatic system. Chemokines are a group of small chemical signals that play an important role in both inflammation and telling immune cells in the bloodstream where to go. They are like special chemical traffic signals. Chemokine mediated lymphatic invasion by cancer cells has been shown to be important in thyroid cancer (Mitchell and Parangi 2005).

Of course both patients and their doctors want to know how we can use this step-by-step knowledge to attack and to kill cancer cells so they don't cause harm to patients. It almost seems we have many pieces of the puzzle, now we just need to put it all together and solve the puzzle. Remember transformation of a normal thyroid cell into a cancerous cell involves many steps, some genetic, some environmental, and some tissue specific. The study of thyroid cancer cells sometimes needs to recapitulate how these steps occur. In order to develop new cures for thyroid cancers, physicians and scientists must be able to study these tumors in controlled laboratory conditions in a way that accurately reproduces the diseases that develop in humans. For every patient with thyroid cancer, the main objective of their physician is to cure the disease with the best available treatments (for example, surgery and radioiodine for thyroid cancer). However, despite fairly good therapies, some thyroid cancers will recur and even become deadly. For these patients, physicians and researchers are working on what causes thyroid cancer to develop resistance to conventional therapies and develop new ways to stop thyroid cancer cells from growing or metastatsizing.

Personal Notes: Learning from Experience
Comments from a Thyroid Researcher

Carmelo Nucera, who has his M.D. and a Ph.D. degree, is an endocrinologist and an instructor at Harvard Medical School. He does basic research on various aspects of thyroid diseases including the regulation of thyroid hormone during fetal development and thyroid cancer development and thyroid tumorigenesis. Originally from Italy, he now lives in Boston with his fiancé Carmen. He writes a personal note about how he managed to get where he is and what sparked his interest in the field of thyroid research:

After finishing medical school in Italy, I went onto a residency in endocrinology and metabolic diseases at the University of Messina in Italy. One day I was asked to see a 19-year-old suffering from a learning disability, obesity, hypoparathyroidism, metabolic syndrome, and severe skin and blood vessel changes. He was a mystery and through some reading and detective work, I managed to figure out that he had a very rare genetic disorder called DiGeorge syndrome. Once the mystery was solved, we started treating the young patient with anti-thrombotic drugs and prevented further damage to the blood vessels to his brain. His family was very happy, to say the least, and appreciated my contribution to the health of their son. After this, I decided to study endocrinology and metabolism and was turned onto the need for research.

While a clinical fellow at Catholic University in Rome, my research lead to the development of a new transgenic animal model to help investigate how thyroid hormone action affects early and late fetal development.

I started thinking about thyroid cancer and was excited to link thyroid cancers with a particular mutation in the B-Raf^{V600E} gene to areas of Sicily rich in volcanic ash. I moved from Italy to Harvard Medical School to pursue research on the importance of this particular gene mutation in the aggressive behavior of thyroid cancer in some people. Being away from my own country and my family has been hard. My work is not complete, but I have managed to publish some excellent results in prestigious journals such as the *Proceedings of the National Academy of Medicine* and this makes all the sacrifices seem worthwhile.

I will never forget the extraordinary scientists that I have met at Harvard Medical School: great persons, great science and education, great everything … Well, I have made many sacrifices in my working life, sacrificing often my private life. I have learned that honesty, hard work, and perseverance are all important factors in doing successful research but these factors are not enough. My family been fantastic in helping me back up when there have been difficult steps in my life. Furthermore, I have been super lucky to meet a stellar woman Carmen who is now my fiancé. She is an oncologist who also studies cancer cells and a fantastic person with super-intelligence and humanity. Her kind, caring, sweet, unselfish personality has helped me make it through the hard times. Doing research makes me happy because I have hope that my scientific discoveries will help patients with thyroid diseases.

Let's look in detail at some of the scientific approaches to blocking tumor angiogenesis within tumors which are currently being developed for patients with thyroid cancer and starting to be tested. Here we are only highlighting this one area because we feel that looking at one research strategy allows you to realize the complexities of the research strategies necessary to even block one little part of the cancer cell's complicated quest for growth. Blocking blood vessel growth in order to block the growth of a tumor is a very new concept. Not so long ago the scientist who first proposed it, Dr. Judah Folkman was ridiculed and told that blocking tumor angiogenesis was crazy. It was thought to be "a pie in the sky" idea. Folkman was a pediatric surgeon and a scientist who in 1971, wrote a seminal article in the prestigious *The New England Journal of Medicine* (Folkman 1971) that all cancerous tumors were dependent on the recruitment of new blood vessels-angiogenesis. If a tumor could be stopped from recruiting and growing its own blood supply, he gathered, it would eventually wither and die. At that time, cancer researchers were focused on killing the actual cancer cells, with anything they could get their hands on, chemotherapy, radiation, and various other agents. This new proposal to kill cancer cells by depriving them of nutrients and oxygen seemed just a little bizarre, especially since it might hurt normal blood vessels in the body and wasn't even aimed at the main culprits, the cancerous cells themselves. Though his hypothesis was initially disregarded by most experts in the field, Folkman persisted with his research. After more than a decade, his theory became widely accepted. First, he concentrated on preventing benign, but sometimes life threatening tangles of blood vessels called *hemangiogmas* which are fairly common problem in infants and children, using a compound found naturally in the body called *interferon*. From there, his research led to the development of progressively more potent compounds, such as angiostatin, endostatin, and vasculostatin, that have successfully halted the growth of tumors in laboratory mice (Folkman 1997). At least 50 angiogenesis inhibitors—including endostatin, angiostatin, 2ME2 (Panzem), and a thrombospondin analogue—are in clinical trials today for cancer treatment, including a number with unanticipated anti-angiogenic effects. These include the anti-inflammatory drug celecoxib (Celebrex); rosiglitazone (Avandia), a drug commonly used to treat type 2 diabetes; doxycycline, a common antibiotic; and some cancer drugs that also have other mechanisms of action, including some traditional chemotherapy drugs. Folkman envisioned that someday, angiogenesis inhibitors would be used together or in combination with conventional anticancer therapies such as chemotherapy, radiotherapy, immunotherapy, gene therapy, or vaccine therapy. Well, Folkman unfortunately died in 2008 before all his pioneering and original thoughts had come to full fruition. However, before he died, he could tell that his groundbreaking predictions had been exactly right, as he got to see a rush of scientist, physicians, pharmaceutical companies, and biotechnology companies joining efforts to launch numerous clinical trials to test combinations of these agents hoping to get the best results for patients with cancer with the least toxicity possible.

Let's get some details here about strategies aimed at the tumor's blood supply. Novel tactics used by scientist to block new blood vessel growth in thyroid cancer include:

1. Blockage of production or activation of angiogenesis stimulators produced by the tumor cells.
2. Stimulation of endogenous inhibitors of angiogenesis.
3. Administration of inhibitors of angiogenesis (*antiangiogenic agents*), for example administration of agents, which cause inhibition of proliferation, chemotaxis, or migration of tumor endothelial cells. Avastin is a good example of a very novel agent directed at inhibiting the growth of new tumor blood vessels.
4. Agents that destroy existing tumor blood vessels—vascular targeting agents. Vascular targeting agents differ conceptually from antiangiogenic agents in that while antiangiogenic agents aim to stop the formation of

One More Thing to Know: Now That's Interesting
A Research Success Story Decades in the Making
Vascular Endothelial Growth Factor (VEGF)

Here is the story of how the discovery of one molecule, secreted by cancer cells to recruit new blood vessels and make them leakier led to one of the most expensive and novel drugs ever developed for cancer therapy in the United States. In 1983, a protein was identified by Dr. Donald Senger which induced blood vessels to become more permeable—that is more porous and leaky, this new factor was called named Vascular Permeability Factor (VPF) (Senger, Perruzzi et al. 1986). It was later discovered that this special chemical signal produced by some cells also caused blood vessels cells to divide and grow, thus the protein also became known as vascular endothelial growth factor (VEGF-A) (Leung, Cachianes et al. 1989). This important protein is believed to regulate the formation of new blood vessels during embryonic development as well as angiogenesis in the adult by its ability to act as a regulator of virtually all the important molecular steps required for forming a new blood vessel. After years of research, additional members of the VEGF family were identified including VEGF-B, VEGF-C, VEGF-D, placental growth factor (PLGF), and endocrine gland-derived vascular endothelial growth factor (EG-VEGF). Of these, VEGF-C has been found to be unique in that its actions are primarily involved in lymphangiogenesis. Soon it became clear that these molecules all contribute tremendously to the recruitment of new blood vessels by cancers.

As suggested by Dr. Judah Folkman 1971, many scientist and pharmaceutical companies started working on this strategy feverishly (Folkman 1971). At first it seemed like a daunting task, but soon enough scientists at Genentech (now this company is called Genenetech/Roche) started focusing targeting the receptors on the surface of endothelial cells. There are two special receptors on the surface of endothelial cells for VEGF, these are called VEGFR1 (or flt-1) and VEGFR2 (or flk-1, KDR), which bind VEGF with a very high affinity. A special mouse was genetically engineered to lack VEGFR1, studies of this important mouse showed that lack of this one receptor resulted in early embryonic death due to lack of malformation of the developing vasculature, suggesting that VEGF action through the VEGFR1 receptor was critical for proper development of new blood vessels. Genenetech researchers were the first to develop a genetically engineered version of a mouse antibody that contains both human and mouse components, Bevacizumab (Avastin) (Ferrara, Hillan et al. 2004). Avastin was the first commercially made angiogenesis inhibitor made to treat cancer by preventing the tumor cells from recruiting new blood vessels and thus nutrients. Genentech is able to produce the antibody in production-scale quantities. This new drug gained approval in 2004 for combination use with standard chemotherapy for metastatic colon cancer and some kinds of kidney cancer. It is now also used in some forms of breast cancer and is undergoing clinical testing in patients with difficult to treat cancers (Welch, Spithoff et al. 2009). Bevacizumab, however, controversially remains one of the most expensive drugs on the market, costing $50,000–100,000 per patient, and some insurance companies have refused to cover the costs. In 2008, sales of Avastin exceeded $2.5 billion (10-K 1 form10-k_2008 .htm GENENTECH 2008).

new blood vessels in tumors, vascular targeting agents aim to destroy existing tumor vessels. Vascular targeting agents cause a characteristic central necrosis of the tumor by exploiting pathophysiologic differences between normal and tumor endothelial cells (Thorpe 2004). Vascular targeting agents can be small molecules such as Combrestatin A4 P (CAP4), which aims to destroy the required tubulin cytoskeleton in rapidly proliferating and immature tumor endothelial cells resulting in cell death.

5. Ligand-directed vascular targeting strategies include using agents that bind selectively to components unique to tumor blood vessels. The target is usually an antibody or peptide directed against a marker that is selectively present in tumor blood vessels but not in the normal blood vessels found in normal thyroid. Targeting these unique moieties can lead to thrombosis of tumor vessels, endothelial cell death, induce changes in shape of endothelial cells, or redirect host defenses to attack tumor endothelium (Davidoff, Ng et al. 2005). One downside to the tumor blood vessel targeting strategies is that all currently identified markers of tumor endothelium are also found on vessels in sites of inflammation, tissue remodeling, and physiologic angiogenesis, just at a lower level. This can mean fairly significant bystander damage to organs that are either undergoing healing or have some inflammation.

Many antiangiogenic treatments have been devised and some look to combine these strategies by carefully looking at the molecular mechanisms of some of the agents. Unfortunately, understanding of the varied mechanisms by which many of the proangiogenic and antiangiogenic agents exert their intracellular effects is still in its infancy. Most studies on treatment of thyroid malignancies with antiangiogenic and vascular targeting agents are in animals. Some *gene therapy* approaches where genes meant to counteract angiogenesis are being brought into thyroid cancer cells by special viruses are also starting to be used, at least in the laboratory (Spitzweg and Morris 2004).

BASIC LABORATORY RESEARCH IN THYROID CANCER: FROM MICE TO MEN

Studying cancer cells in isolation in a dish (*in vitro*, Latin, "in glass") is helpful to understand important factors involved in how thyroid cancers cells grow and develop. Unfortunately, however, this method does not fully reproduce the biologic behavior of the cancer as we see it in our patients. As an example of this, some thyroid cancer cell lines grow slowly in a Petri dish but produce invasive and lethal tumors when injected into a mouse. Conversely, other cell lines grow rapidly *in vitro* but have little ability to develop as tumors when injected into the thyroid gland of an animal. A likely explanation for this disparity of behavior is that cancers develop and grow in tissues and organs with a complex surrounding environment rather than in isolation. In the thyroid gland, for example, the cancers that develop are surrounded by thyroid follicular cells, colloid, surrounding stroma, and are fed by a blood supply that delivers the components of the body's immune system. So to study cancers only using *in vitro* techniques is like studying the behavior of a fish in a glass bowl rather than in the open ocean: it fails to account for the myriad factors of the environment that can influence its behavior.

Animal models of cancer can help overcome this limitation. In the simplest animal models, tumor cells are injected under the skin (*subcutaneously*) of mouse with a defective immune system (*immunocompromised mouse*), and the tumor is allowed to grow. This method is popular with researchers because it is technically simple, takes relatively little time to perform, and it allows for easy tumor measurement. The downside of this technique is that there are some natural compounds in skin tissue that prevent the growth and metastasis of cancer cells, which skews the scientist's ability to test and understand how cancer behaves in its native location.

A better way to reproduce the biology of human cancers is by using an *orthotopic* model ("orthotopic means into the organ of origin such as the thyroid"). In these animal models, human thyroid cancer cells are directly injected into the organ of origin with a small operation to deliver the cells into the thyroid. The cancer cells can grow and develop in the native environment in order to reproduce the kind of disease we are trying to treat. For example, in a mouse model of the very aggressive 'anaplastic' thyroid cancer, mice develop large and invasive neck tumors with numerous metastases to the lungs. This is an accurate representation of how the disease behaves in humans and allows scientists to test new drugs and other therapies against these aggressive diseases. This model, however, is more technically challenging and more expensive compared with subcutaneous models.

A third type of animal cancer model is called *transgenic* or *genetically engineered* model. In this type of experiment, foreign cancer-causing genes can be inserted into the DNA of an embryonic mouse that will cause the mouse to develop thyroid cancer later in its life. The first transgenic model of cancer was developed by Dr. Douglas Hanahan in 1985 (Hanahan 1985). His model focused on over expressing a cancer gene specifically in the insulin producing cells of the mouse pancreas and fairly quickly the mice developed a rare cancer called *Insulinoma*. Every single mouse developed the same tumor and within a few weeks, the mice would die. This was the first time a gene had been manipulated in a mouse and led to cancer. It was pretty revolutionary and soon enough researchers started developing similar transgenic mouse models of thyroid cancer by manipulating various genes known to be important in thyroid cancer (Santoro, Chiappetta et al. 1996; Powell, Russell et al. 1998; Knauf, Ma et al. 2005). This type of model is perhaps the best representation of thyroid cancer in humans because the tumor develops from the thyroid tissue of the mouse rather than from an injection of cultured human cancer cells. The drawbacks to this type of experiment include increased cost, technically difficult genetic manipulations, and significant time to develop the model.

Although most patients with thyroid cancer can be effectively treated with our standard treatments, some patients will develop recurrences, metastases, and die of their disease. For these patients, scientist and physicians are hard at work to improve the knowledge of their diseases to arrive at new and useful treatments. While *in vitro* studies are immensely helpful in understanding the molecular nature of these cancers, animal models are the best way to test and validate new therapies to demonstrate both safety and efficacy prior to human use. Physicians and scientists must balance the important factors of time, costs, and similarity of the model to its human disease counterpart when deciding which animal model is most appropriate. With the use of these animal models, new and perhaps targeted treatments for aggressive thyroid cancers are sure to be discovered.

REFERENCES

10-K 1 form10-k_2008.htm GENENTECH, I. F. K. F. T. P. E. D., 2008 (2008). "10K forms Genentech Inc in 2008." www.sec.gov/Archives/edgar/data/318771/000031877109000003/form10-k_2008.htm.

Danko, M. E. and M. A. Skinner (2006). "Surgical intervention in children with multiple endocrine neoplasia type 2." *Curr Opin Pediatr* **18**(3): 312–15.

Davidoff, A. M., C. Y. Ng, et al. (2005). "Careful decoy receptor titering is required to inhibit tumor angiogenesis while avoiding adversely altering VEGF bioavailability." *Mol Ther* **11**(2): 300–10.

Durante, C., E. Puxeddu, et al. (2007). "BRAF mutations in papillary thyroid carcinomas inhibit genes involved in iodine metabolism." *J Clin Endocrinol Metab* **92**(7): 2840–43.

Ferrara, N., K. J. Hillan, et al. (2004). "Discovery and development of bevacizumab, an anti-VEGF antibody for treating cancer." *Nat Rev Drug Discov* **3**(5): 391–400.

Folkman, J. (1971). "Tumor angiogenesis: therapeutic implications." *N Engl J Med* **285**(21): 1182–86.

Folkman, J. (1992). "The role of angiogenesis in tumor growth." *Semin Cancer Biol* **3**(2): 65–71.

Folkman, J. (1996). "Fighting cancer by attacking its blood supply." *Sci Am* **275**(3): 150–54.

Folkman, J. (1997). "Angiogenesis and angiogenesis inhibition: an overview." *Exs* **79**: 1–8.

Hanahan, D. (1985). "Heritable formation of pancreatic beta-cell tumours in transgenic mice expressing recombinant insulin/simian virus 40 oncogenes." *Nature* **315**(6015): 115–22.

Iruela-Arispe, M. L. and H. F. Dvorak (1997). "Angiogenesis: a dynamic balance of stimulators and inhibitors." *Thromb Haemost* **78**(1): 672–77.

Knauf, J. A., X. Ma, et al. (2005). "Targeted expression of BRAFV600E in thyroid cells of transgenic mice results in papillary thyroid cancers that undergo dedifferentiation." *Cancer Research* **65**(10): 4238–45.

Kurihara, T., S. Ikeda, et al. (2004). "Immunohistochemical and sequencing analyses of the Wnt signaling components in Japanese anaplastic thyroid cancers." *Thyroid* **14**(12): 1020–29.

Leung, D. W., G. Cachianes, et al. (1989). "Vascular endothelial growth factor is a secreted angiogenic mitogen." *Science* **246**(4935): 1306–9.

Liu, Z., P. Hou, et al. (2008). "Highly prevalent genetic alterations in receptor tyrosine kinases and phosphatidylinositol 3-kinase/akt and mitogen-activated protein kinase pathways in anaplastic and follicular thyroid cancers." *J Clin Endocrinol Metab* **93**(8): 3106–16.

Lui, W. O., T. Foukakis, et al. (2005). "Expression profiling reveals a distinct transcription signature in follicular thyroid carcinomas with a PAX8-PPAR(gamma) fusion oncogene." *Oncogene* **24**(8): 1467–76.

Mitchell, J. C. and S. Parangi (2005). "Angiogenesis in benign and malignant thyroid disease." *Thyroid* **15**(6): 494–510.

Nikiforov, Y. E. (2004). "Genetic alterations involved in the transition from well-differentiated to poorly differentiated and anaplastic thyroid carcinomas." *Endocr Pathol* **15**(4): 319–27.

Powell, D. J., Jr., J. Russell, et al. (1998). "The RET/PTC3 oncogene: metastatic solid-type papillary carcinomas in murine thyroids." *Cancer Res* **58**(23): 5523–28.

Read, A. P. and T. Strachan (1999). Chapter 18: *Cancer Genetics . . . Human molecular genetics 2*. New York, Wiley.

Sanso, G. E., H. M. Domene, et al. (2002). "Very early detection of RET proto-oncogene mutation is crucial for preventive thyroidectomy in multiple endocrine neoplasia type 2 children: presence of C-cell malignant disease in asymptomatic carriers." *Cancer* **94**(2): 323–30.

Santoro, M., G. Chiappetta, et al. (1996). "Development of thyroid papillary carcinomas secondary to tissue-specific expression of the RET/PTC1 oncogene in transgenic mice." *Oncogene* **12**(8): 1821–26.

Schlumberger, M. J., R. Elisei, et al. (2009). "Phase II study of safety and efficacy of motesanib in patients with progressive or symptomatic, advanced or metastatic medullary thyroid cancer." *J Clin Oncol* **27**(23): 3794–801.

Senger, D. R., C. A. Perruzzi, et al. (1986). "A highly conserved vascular permeability factor secreted by a variety of human and rodent tumor cell lines." *Cancer Res* **46**(11): 5629–32.

Spitzweg, C. and J. C. Morris (2004). "Gene therapy for thyroid cancer: current status and future prospects." *Thyroid* **14**(6): 424–34.

Szinnai, G., S. Sarnacki, et al. (2007). "Hereditary medullary thyroid carcinoma: how molecular genetics made multiple endocrine neoplasia type 2 a paediatric disease." *Endocr Dev* **10**: 173–87.

Thorpe, P. E. (2004). "Vascular targeting agents as cancer therapeutics." *Clin Cancer Res* **10**(2): 415–27.

Tjio, H. J. L., A. Levan, (1956). "The chromosome numbers of man." *Hereditas* **42**: 1–6.

Trask, B. J. (2002). "Human cytogenetics: 46 chromosomes, 46 years and counting." *Nat Rev Genet* **3**(10): 769–78.

Welch, S., K. Spithoff, et al. (2010). "Bevacizumab combined with chemotherapy for patients with advanced colorectal cancer: a systematic review." *Ann Oncol.* **21**(6): 1152–62.

Wells, S. A., Jr. and M. Santoro (2009). "Targeting the RET pathway in thyroid cancer." *Clin Cancer Res* **15**(23): 7119–23.

Xing, M., W. H. Westra, et al. (2005). "BRAF mutation predicts a poorer clinical prognosis for papillary thyroid cancer." *J Clin Endocrinol Metab* **90**(12): 6373–79.

Resources and Organizations

The American Association of Clinical Endocrinologists (AACE)

245 Riverside Ave, Suite 200
Jacksonville, FL 32202
(904) 353-7878
Web: www.aace.com

The American Association of Clinical Endocrinologists is a professional community of physicians specializing in endocrinology, diabetes, and metabolism committed to enhancing the ability of its members to provide the highest quality of patient care. Their Web site lists their organizational overview as:

> Members of AACE are physicians with special education, training, and interest in the practice of clinical endocrinology. These physicians devote a significant part of their career to the evaluation and management of patients with endocrine disease. All members of AACE are physicians (M.D. or D.O.) and a majority is certified by Boards recognized by the American Board of Medical Specialties. Members of AACE are recognized clinicians, educators and scientists, many of whom are affiliated with medical schools and universities. Members of AACE contribute on a regular and continuing basis to the

scientific literature on endocrine diseases and conduct medical education programs on this subject.

American Association of Endocrine Surgeons

5810 W. 140th Terrace
Overland Park, KS 66223
(913) 402-7102
Fax: (913) 273-9940
E-mail:information@endocrinesurgery.org
Web: www.endocrinesurgery.org

The American Association of Endocrine Surgeons (AAES) is a representative body of surgeons from North America, South America and Mexico who have a special interest in the surgery of endocrine glands. This Association was established in 1981 and continues to grow and expand its membership to include corresponding members (endocrine surgeons from other countries throughout the world), honorary members (physicians outside the discipline of surgery who have contributed significantly to the field of endocrine surgical disease) and allied health members (otolaryngologists, urologists, neurosurgeons, etc. who have acquired considerable expertise in the field of endocrine surgery). The goals and objectives of the AAES are to enhance the advancement of the science and the art of endocrine surgery. The Association is also dedicated to the maintenance of high standards in the practice of endocrine surgery. The AAES is committed to providing surgical expertise in diseases of the thyroid, parathyroid, adrenal glands as well as in neuroendocrine tumors of the pancreas and GI tract. Their goal is to discover and promote the best treatments for endocrine disease to help improve our patients' lives. The AAES maintains an impressive, accurate and detailed patient education site.

The American Thyroid Association (ATA)

American Thyroid Association
6066 Leesburg Pike, Suite 550
Falls Church, VA 22041
E-mail: thyroid@thyroid.org
Web: www.thyroid.org

The ATA is a leader in promoting thyroid health and understanding thyroid biology. The ATA is an important organization focused on thyroid biology and the prevention and treatment of thyroid disorders through excellence and innovation in research. Important goals of the ATA are listed on their Web site and includes:

1. To foster and support research on thyroid molecular and cell biology, physiology, and diseases.
2. To disseminate new knowledge that leads to prevention, diagnosis, and treatment of thyroid diseases.
3. To support education of trainees, basic scientists, physicians, and other health care professionals concerned with investigating, diagnosing, and treating thyroid diseases.
4. To establish and guide public policies on the causes, diagnosis, and management of thyroid diseases and related disorders.
5. To be the advocate for thyroid specialists in the councils concerned with science, clinical medicine, and health care delivery.
6. To encourage broad-based support from industry and other parties to fulfill the association's scientific and educational missions.
7. To stimulate philanthropic giving to a fund that supports the association's activities.
8. To enlarge and diversify the association's membership.
9. To develop, implement, and regularly review the association's long-term plan.
10. To foster contact, collegiality, and collaboration among members and within the international thyroid community.
11. To promote collaboration with thyroid societies in other regions of the world concerning public health and other scientific issues.

National Cancer Institute (NCI)

NCI Public Inquiries Office
Suite 3036A
6116 Executive Boulevard, MSC8322
Bethesda, MD 20892-8322
(800) 422-6237
Web: www.cancer.gov

The National Cancer Institute (NCI) is part of the National Institutes of Health (NIH), which is one of 11 agencies that compose the U.S. Department of Health and Human Services (HHS). The NCI, established under the National Cancer Institute Act of 1937, is the Federal Government's principal agency for cancer research and training. The National Cancer Act of 1971 broadened the scope and responsibilities of the NCI and created the National Cancer Program. Over the years, legislative amendments have maintained the NCI authorities and responsibilities and added new information dissemination mandates as well as a requirement to assess the incorporation of state-of-the-art cancer treatments into clinical practice.

The National Cancer Institute coordinates the National Cancer Program, which conducts and supports research, training, health information dissemination, and other programs with respect to the cause, diagnosis, prevention, and treatment of cancer, rehabilitation from cancer, and the continuing care of cancer patients and the families of cancer patients. Specifically, the Institute:

1. Supports and coordinates research projects conducted by universities, hospitals, research foundations, and businesses throughout this country and abroad through research grants and cooperative agreements.
2. Conducts research in its own laboratories and clinics.
3. Supports education and training in fundamental sciences and clinical disciplines for participation in basic and clinical research programs and treatment programs relating to cancer through career awards, training grants, and fellowships.
4. Supports research projects in cancer control.
5. Supports a national network of cancer centers.
6. Collaborates with voluntary organizations and other national and foreign institutions engaged in cancer research and training activities.
7. Encourages and coordinates cancer research by industrial concerns where such concerns evidence a particular capability for programmatic research.
8. Collects and disseminates information on cancer.
9. Supports construction of laboratories, clinics, and related facilities necessary for cancer research through the award of construction grants.

National Library of Medicine (NLM)

National Library of Medicine
8600 Rockville Pike
Bethesda, MD 20894
(888) 346-3656
(301) 594-5983
Web: www.nlm.nih.gov/

NLM in Bethesda, Maryland, is a part of the National Institutes of Health, U.S. Department of Health and Human Services (HHS). Since its founding in 1836, NLM has played a pivotal role in translating biomedical research into practice. It is the world's largest biomedical library and the developer of electronic information services that deliver trillions of bytes of data to millions of users every day. Scientists, health professionals, and the public in the United States and around the globe search the library's online information resources more than one billion times each year.

The library is open to all and has many services and resources—for scientists, health professionals, historians, and the general public. NLM has nearly 12 million books, journals, manuscripts, audiovisuals, and other forms of medical information on its shelves, making it the largest health-science library in the world.

In today's increasingly digital world, NLM carries out its mission of enabling biomedical research, supporting health care and public health, and promoting healthy behavior by:

1. Acquiring, organizing, and preserving the world's scholarly biomedical literature.
2. Providing access to biomedical and health information across the country in partnership with the 5,600-member National Network of Libraries of Medicine (NN/LM®).
3. Serving as a leading global resource for building, curating, and providing sophisticated access to molecular biology and genomic information, including those from the Human Genome Project and NIH Roadmap.
4. Creating high quality information services relevant to toxicology and environmental health, health services research, and public health.
5. Conducting research and development on biomedical communications systems, methods, technologies, and networks and information dissemination and utilization among health professionals, patients, and the general public.
6. Funding advanced biomedical informatics research and serving as the primary supporter of pre- and post-doctoral research training in biomedical informatics at 18 U.S. universities.

The Endocrine Society

8401 Connecticut Ave., Suite 900
Chevy Chase, MD 20815
(888) 363-6274
(301) 941-0200
Web: www.endo-society.org

The Endocrine Society's stated mission is "to advance excellence in endocrinology and promote its essential role as an integrative force in scientific research and medical practice." Among its goals, the society aims to "emphasize the integration of the field and the importance of basic research and its translation to patient care."

ThyCa: Thyroid Cancer Survivor Association Inc.

P.O. Box 1545
New York, NY 10159-1545
(877) 588-7904
Web: www.thyca.org

ThyCa is "a national non-profit 501(c)(3) organization (tax ID #52-2169434) of thyroid cancer survivors, family members, and health care professionals. They are dedicated to support, education, and communication for thyroid cancer survivors, their families, and friends. They also sponsor Thyroid Cancer Awareness Month, year-round awareness activities, and thyroid cancer research fundraising and research grants. This site maintains current information about thyroid cancer and support services available to people at any stage of testing, treatment, or lifelong monitoring for thyroid cancer, as well as their caregivers. It receives ongoing input and review from numerous thyroid cancer specialists. This site also serves as a resource for anyone interested in thyroid cancer survivors' issues."
    ThyCa describes its mission as:

To educate, so patients and families better understand thyroid cancer.
To participate, so others learn from our experience.
To communicate, so patients and health care professionals better understand each others' needs.
To support research for a future free of thyroid cancer.

Endocrine Nurses Society

P.O. Box 211068
Milwaukee WI 53221
(414) 421-3679
Web: www.endo-nurses.org

A society for supporting nursing research related to the care of patients with endocrine disorders. The Endocrine Nurses Society describes itself as "a professional organization for endocrine nurses founded to promote excellence in the clinical care of patients through advancement of the science and art of endocrine nursing."

Glossary

Agranulocytosis: A medical condition in which there is a sudden and severe and dangerous drop in the white blood cell count, especially of the kind most active in fighting infection—the neutrophils. Agranulocytosis may involve more sub-types of white blood cells. People with this condition are at very high risk of serious infections due to suppression of their immune system. Thionamides which are sometimes used to treat hyperthyroidism can rarely lead to this potentially fatal complication.

Albumin: A common water-soluble protein coagulated by heat found in blood plasma. Serum albumin is the most abundant protein in the blood and is produced in the liver. Albumin helps chaperone many other less soluble proteins in the blood and thus is sometimes called "the molecular taxi." It does also help chaperone thyroid hormone in the bloodstream to important destinations throughout the body.

Anaplastic thyroid carcinoma: A form of thyroid cancer with a very poor prognosis and a very low ten year survival rate compared to other forms of thyroid cancers. Anaplastic thyroid carcinoma grows very rapidly and spreads through direct invasion of surrounding structures. These structures include the trachea and/or recurrent laryngeal nerve, and also the esophagus, jugular veins, and carotid arteries. Unfortunately, anaplastic thyroid carcinoma also forms metastases early on, and 50–60 percent of people with anaplastic thyroid carcinoma already have distant metastases to lungs, bone, and brain at the time of diagnosis.

Anesthesia: Having sensation including the feeling of pain blocked or temporarily taken away by using special chemical agents called anesthetics. This allows patients to undergo surgery and other procedures without the distress and pain they would otherwise experience. Anesthesia is a pharmacologically induced reversible state of amnesia, analgesia, loss of responsiveness, loss of skeletal muscle reflexes, and decreased stress response.

Angiogenesis: Physiologic process by which new blood vessels are formed from old blood vessels. This is a fundamental step in the transition of tumors from a slow growing or benign state to a malignant one. The balance between stimulators and inhibitors of angiogenesis is a tightly regulated process that allows for no angiogenesis in normal adult tissues. Once this balance is disturbed, either through an increase in stimulatory signals or a decrease in inhibitory signals, then angiogenesis will begin. Stimulators of angiogenesis are special factors often produced by the cancer cells themselves that turn on angiogenesis and cause active recruitment of new blood vessels. A class of drugs called antiangiogenic agents have been developed that try to suppress angiogenesis in a variety of diseases including heart disease, macular degeneration, arthritis, and cancer.

Antiangiogenic agent: A substance that actively inhibits the process by which new blood vessels form from old blood vessels. Many antiangiogenic agents which are also known as angiogenesis inhibitors are currently being developed and tested for use in humans with cancer.

Anti-Thyroglobulin Antibodies: Autoimmune antibodies present in some patients with autoimmune thyroid disease that attack thyroglobulin. If present in the bloodstream they will interfere with accuracy of blood tests that measure thyroglobulin levels. If a person has thyroglobulin antibodies then thyroglobulin levels cannot be used to track tumor growth.

Anti-Thyroid Peroxidase Antibodies: Autoimmune antibodies present in some patients with autoimmune thyroid disorders, especially those with autoimmune hypothyroidism. These antibodies attack the special enzyme in the thyroid that processes iodine into thyroid hormone—thyroid peroxidase. High thyroid peroxidase antibody level usually predicts mild to moderate thyroid dysfunction and signal the fact that the thyroid may be on its way to burning out from autoimmune hypothyroidism.

Anti-TSH Receptor Antibodies: Autoimmune antibodies present in some patients with autoimmune hyperthyroidism. These antibodies constantly stimulate the thyroid by docking into the receptor for TSH and deceiving the thyroid into constant stimulation. This condition is called Graves' disease and these antibodies mimic the action of TSH which is normally regulated by the pituitary. These antibodies, however, have gone awry and result in constant stimulation of the thyroid and results in severe hyperthyroidism. Finding this particular antibody in high quantity in the serum is indicative of Graves' disease and rarely other forms of autoimmune thyroiditis.

Benign: A condition where a tumor is present but lacks all three of the malignant properties of a cancer. Thus, by definition, a benign tumor does not grow in an unlimited, aggressive manner, does not invade surrounding tissues or organs and does not spread (metastasize) to non-adjacent tissues. Some thyroid nodules are benign tumors. Some neoplasms which are defined as "benign tumors" because they lack the invasive properties of cancer, may still produce negative health effects.

Biopsy: A medical test involving the removal of cells or tissue samples for examination to determine the presence or extent of a disease. The tissue is generally examined under a microscope by a pathologist, and can also be analyzed chemically or for genetic changes. When an entire lump or suspicious area is removed, the procedure is called an *excisional biopsy*. When only a sample of tissue is removed with preservation of the architecture of the tissue's cells, the procedure is called an *incisional biopsy* or *core biopsy*. When a sample of tissue or fluid is removed with a needle in such a way that cells are removed without preserving the histological architecture of the tissue cells, the procedure is called a *fine needle aspiration biopsy*.

Calcifications: The process in which calcium salts build up in soft tissue, causing it to harden. Calcifications seen on thyroid ultrasound can sometimes be a sign of thyroid cancer especially if they are very tiny.

Calcitonin: A 32-amino acid linear polypeptide hormone produced by the parafollicular cells (also known as C-cells) of the thyroid. In humans its function is usually not very significant but it is thought to reduce blood calcium levels (Ca^{2+}), opposing the effects of parathyroid hormone (PTH).

Cancer: A class of diseases in which a group of cells display *uncontrolled growth* beyond the normal limits, invasion and destruction of adjacent tissues, and sometime metastasis or spread to other locations in the body via lymph or blood. The branch of medicine concerned with the study, diagnosis, treatment, and prevention of cancer is oncology. Thyroid cancer is often, however, treated by endocrinologists and not oncologists.

Carotid artery: A large artery on each side of the neck that supplies blood to the head, neck and brain. The carotid artery gives off the main blood supply to the thyroid.

Chemokine: Are a family of small special cytokines or proteins secreted by cells that act to create a chemical attraction to nearby responsive cells. They act as a chemoattractant to guide the migration of cells and different ones help with guiding immune or inflammatory cells to sites of infection such as lymph nodes, but can also be key molecules in guiding cancer cells into lymph nodes.

Colloid: Serves as a reservoir of materials for thyroid hormone production and, to a lesser extent, act as a reservoir for the hormones themselves. Colloid is rich in a protein called thyroglobulin.

Computed Axial Tomography (CAT scan): A radiologic imaging modality that uses ionizing radiation and powerful computers to obtain precise thin cut images of the body, including the neck and thyroid gland. CAT scans are rarely used as a first tool in imaging the thyroid, since it is not very good at discerning differences between benign and cancerous growths in the thyroid. This test is very good at looking for enlarged thyroid goiters that are substernal in location or in those with very large cancers which may be attached to other nearby organs.

Conception: The process by which an embryo is made when of an ovum from the female is fused with a sperm from the male.

Cretinism: A condition associated with congenital hypothyroidism or iodine deficiency which results in lower intelligence levels. Cretinism is a form of hypothyroidism found in infants.

Deoiodinase: These selenium containing enzymes are important in the activation and inactivation of thyroid hormone through the removal of an iodine atom from the inner or outer ring of thyroid hormone. Three catalyzing enzymes have been identified, called type 1 (D1), type 2 (D2), and type 3 (D3).

Ectopic thyroid tissue: A developmental defect in the fetus can lead to pieces of thyroid tissue being left along the track the thyroid takes during its descent from its original location at the base of the tongue.

Endemic goiter: Goiter that is "prevalent in" a particular region, usually due to iodine deficiency or goiterogens. Iodine, a mineral found in seawater, is essential for normal function of the thyroid. Since iodine is essential for the thyroid to make thyroid hormone, a short supply of iodine causes increased TSH, stimulation, and enlargement of the thyroid gland as it tries to compensate. Goiterogens are special chemicals found in certain foods that interfere with the body's ability to properly use iodine to synthesize thyroid hormone.

Endocrine surgeon: Medical doctors who specialize in the diagnosis and treatment of diseases of the endocrine glands which may require surgery, including the thyroid, parathyroid, adrenal, and pancreas. The commonest endocrine surgery operation is removal of the thyroid (thyroidectomy) followed by parathyroid surgery (parathyroidectomy) then more rare operations on the adrenal gland (adrenalectomy). Endocrine surgeon have full training as general surgeons for five years followed by a one to two year fellowship which allows further specialization for removal of tumors from endocrine organs.

Endocrine system: The endocrine system consists of several glands, in different parts of the body that secrete hormones directly into the blood rather than into a duct system. Hormones have many different functions and modes of action; one hormone may have several effects on different target organs, and, conversely, one target organ may be affected by more than one hormone. The thyroid gland is an endocrine organ.

Endocrinologist: Medical doctor who specialize in hormone producing *endocrine* organs such as the thyroid, pituitary, or pancreas. They can order blood tests and imaging tests of the thyroid and can help diagnose these somewhat complex diseases. The medical specialty of endocrinology involves the diagnostic evaluation of a wide variety of symptoms and variations and the long-term management of disorders of deficiency or excess of one or more hormones.

Esophagus: A muscular tube which acts as the passage down which food moves between the throat and the stomach.

Exopthalmus: Bulging of the eyes or orbital space. This condition can be caused by Graves' disease of the thyroid and in some cases can be quite severe.

Fertility: The natural capability of giving life. Infertility is deficient fertility.

Fine needle aspiration (FNA): Removal of a small cluster of cells or fluid from a thyroid nodule using a very small needle attached to a syringe. The aspirated cells are analyzed under a microscope by an experienced *cytologist* (a doctor specializing in pathology who has extra training to look at individual clusters of cells) and categorized as benign or malignant. It is not always possible to make a decision despite accurate or multiple fine needle aspirations. This procedure is safe and can be performed in the office of the physician.

Follicular carcinoma: A type of well-differentiated thyroid cancer and is the second-most common thyroid cancer representing ten percent of all thyroid cancers Follicular carcinoma often presents at a later age and is more common in regions of the world with iodine. Unlike papillary thyroid cancer, follicular carcinoma rarely spreads to the lymph nodes, but can present with direct invasion into anatomical structures adjacent to the thyroid gland or may spread to distant organs via the bloodstream at a significantly higher rate than papillary thyroid.

Gene therapy: A biologic technique whereby genes are inserted into an individual cell or tissue to treat diseases such as cancer or inherited diseases such as sickle cell. Although the technology is still in its infancy, it has been used with some success to replace a mutant gene with a healthy one. Scientific breakthroughs continue to move gene therapy toward mainstream medicine.

Gland: In animals, it is a cell or group of cells that secretes a specific substance. Endocrine glands secrete directly into the bloodstream, while exocrine glands secrete through ducts into a cavity or to the surface of the body. The thyroid is an endocrine gland.

Glucocorticoid steroids: A class of steroid hormones that bind to the glucocorticoid receptor, which is present in almost every vertebrate animal cell. They are produced in the cortex of the adrenal gland. Cortisol or hydrocortisone is the most important human glucocorticoid, and it is essential for life. These hormones are often administered to reduce inflammation.

Goiter: Enlargement of the thyroid gland appearing as a swelling of the front of the neck. Iodine deficiency is one of several causes.

Goiterogens: Special chemicals found in certain foods that interfere with the body's ability to properly use iodine to synthesize thyroid hormone.

Graves' disease: An autoimmune disease in which there is generally enlargement of the thyroid as well as overproduction of thyroid hormone—hyperthyroidism. The changes are caused by auto antibodies to the TSH-eceptor (TSHR-Ab) that activate that TSH-receptor, thereby stimulating thyroid hormone synthesis, secretion, and thyroid growth (causing a diffuse goiter) as well as hormone excess. The resulting state of hyperthyroidism causes a dramatic constellation of neuropsychological and physical signs and symptoms, and has profound effects on the heart and cardiovascular system. Graves' disease is the most common cause of severe hyperthyroidism and is accompanied by impressive clinical signs and symptoms and laboratory abnormalities as compared with milder forms of hyperthyroidism. Graves' disease is sometimes called diffuse toxic goiter because it involves the entire thyroid gland.

Hemostasis: A complex process which causes the bleeding process to stop. It refers to the process of keeping blood within a damaged blood vessel (the opposite of hemostasis is hemorrhage). Hemostasis has three major steps: 1) vasoconstriction, 2) temporary blockage of a break by a platelet plug, and 3) blood coagulation, or formation of a clot that seals the hole until tissue are repaired. Achieving proper hemostasis is an important part of any kind of surgery; this is especially true for thyroid surgery since the thyroid is removed from on top of the trachea.

Homeostasis: The property of regulation in a closed system which allows its internal environment to maintain a stable, constant condition. Multiple dynamic equilibrium adjustment and regulation mechanisms make homeostasis possible.

Hormone: A chemical secreted by an endocrine gland or some nerve cells that regulates the function of a specific tissue or organ.

Human Chorionic Gonadotropin (hCG): A hormone that is important for pregnancy but can stimulate the thyroid gland to produce more thyroid hormone and therefore decrease the amounts of TSH in the blood.

Hürthle cell carcinoma: A rare thyroid cancer that is currently considered a variant of follicular thyroid carcinoma. It is unique from other follicular thyroid carcinomas in that 75–100 percent of the tumor is composed of Hürthle cells. These cells are rotund, polygonal follicular cells that contain abundant cytoplasm, and can be found in a variety of benign thyroid conditions, such as Hashimoto thyroiditis, Graves's disease, and multinodular goiter. Hürthle-cell carcinomas account for two or three percent of all thyroid malignancies and are diagnosed most often in the fifth decade of life. Hürthle-cell carcinomas are significantly more aggressive with a higher likelihood of metastasis to distant organs such as bone.

Hürthle cell: A cell in the thyroid that is often associated with Hashimoto's thyroiditis but can also be seen in some follicular neoplasms such Hürthle cell adenoma or Hürthle cell carcinoma. Hürthle cells are characterized as enlarged epithelial cells with abundant eosinophilic granular cytoplasm as a result of altered mitochondria. They generally stain pink and are quite prominent under the microscope.

Hydatidiform mole: Product of an abnormal pregnancy wherein a non-viable, fertilized egg implants in the uterus, and thereby converts normal pregnancy processes into pathological ones. No identifiable embryonic or fetal tissues arise when an empty egg with no nucleus is fertilized by one (or occasionally two) normal sperm. Hydatidiform moles may develop into choriocarcinoma, a form of cancer, which can be a very rare cause of hyperthyroidism. Some Hydatidiform moles or choriocarcinomas produce large amounts of human chorionic gonadotropin (hCG) a protein normally produced by the placenta during pregnancy. Excessive amounts of hCG can directly bind to the TSH receptors on the thyroid gland and stimulate thyroid hormone release causing hyperthyroidism.

Hyperthyroidism: The term for overactive thyroid tissue causing too much thyroid hormone. Hyperthyroidism is one of the causes of thyrotoxicosis, a clinical condition of increased thyroid hormones in the blood. It is important to note that hyperthyroidism and thyrotoxicosis are not synonymous. For instance, thyrotoxicosis could instead be caused by ingestion of exogenous thyroid hormone or inflammation of the thyroid gland, causing it to release its stores of thyroid hormones. Major clinical signs of hyperthyroidism include weight loss often accompanied by an increased appetite, anxiety, feeling hot, hair loss, muscle aches, weakness, fatigue, hyperactivity, irritability, tremor, and excessive sweating. Additionally, patients may present with a variety of symptoms such as palpitations, irregular heartbeat, shortness of breath, and diarrhea. Often, in the elderly, these classical symptoms may not be present.

Hypothalamus: A tiny gland the size of an almond in the brain that helps regulate many neural and hormonal outputs and responses in the body. The hypothalamus co-ordinates many hormonal and behavioral circadian rhythms, complex patterns of neuroendocrine outputs, complex homeostatic mechanisms, and many other important hormones throughout the body. The hypothalamus makes Thyroid Releasing Hormone (TRH) which is carried down to the pituitary and acts as a signal to increase production of Thyroid Stimulating Hormone (TSH).

Hypothyroidism: Condition in humans when the thyroid gland does not produce sufficient quantities of thyroid hormone. Iodine deficiency is the most common cause of hypothyroidism worldwide. Major clinical signs of hypothyroidism includes: fatigue, cold intolerance, muscle cramps, joint pain, brittle hair, depression, dry itchy skin, weight gain, and constipation.

Immune system: A system of biological structures and processes within an humans and other organisms that protects against diseases by identifying and killing foreign pathogens including viruses and bacteria as well as tumor cells. Disorders in the immune system can result in diseases. Autoimmune diseases result from a hyperactive immune system attacking normal tissues as if they were foreign organisms. Hashimoto's thyroiditis is a common inflammatory autoimmune disease that is caused by antibodies aimed at destroying the thyroid gland.

Immunocompromised: A state in which an animal or a human has a compromised immune system such that fighting infection or tumor cells is very difficult. Immunocompromised mice are commonly used in cancer research because human tumor cells can grow in them due to the defective immune system.

In vitro: Experiments performed in a controlled environment such as a test tube or tissue culture dish and not in a living organism. In vitro experiments are the cornerstone of basic laboratory research in cancer biology. When publishing such experimental results, the annotation is in vitro, in contradistinction with in vivo which means the experiments were conducted in animals.

In vivo: Experiments performed in a whole, living organism as opposed to in a test tube or tissue cultured dish in a controlled laboratory environment. Animal testing of drugs and clinical trials in humans with cancer are two forms of *in vivo* research.

Incidence: A measure of the risk of developing some new condition within a specified period of time.

Insulinoma: A tumor of the pancreas that secretes insulin. These tumors can lead to dangerously low glucose levels and can lead to a state of insulin shock.

Interferon: Proteins made and released by white blood cells in response to the presence of viruses, bacteria, or tumor cells. They have been used as a therapeutic strategy against certain cancers.

Iodine: A poisonous, dark gray to purple-black, lustrous, nonmetallic crystalline element in the halogen family. This element is often used every day in germicide, antiseptic, preparation of dyes, pharmaceuticals, tinctures, isotopes in medicine, and industry. It is a critical element for proper growth and function of the thyroid gland. Iodate, a more stable form of iodine, has been used as an additive to salt in many parts of the world to prevent iodine deficiency in humans worldwide.

Jod-Basedow phenomena: A physiologic phenomena whereby administration of exogenous extra iodine to a person with previously baseline iodine deficiency can trigger severe episodes of hyperthyroidism

Jugular vein: Any one of four pairs of veins in the neck that drain blood from the head, neck, and brain. A larger internal jugular vein is flanked by an external vein on each side of the neck.

Lacrimal ducts: The small channels in each eyelid that allows drainage of tears. Lacrimal ducts can be damaged by radioactive iodine because they contain iodine receptors. Damage to these glands can lead to constant tearing.

Ligature: Consists of a piece of surgical thread or suture tied around an anatomical structure, usually a blood vessel or another hollow structure to shut it off. With a blood vessel the surgeon will clamp the vessel perpendicular to the axis of the artery or vein with a hemostat, then secure it by ligating it i.e., using a piece of suture around it before dividing the structure then releasing the hemostat. Surgical ties can be made of synthetic material such as nylon or natural material such as silk. Silk ties are still commonly used in thyroid surgery.

Lingual thyroid: An anatomic variation or congenital defect where thyroid tissue can remain in its original position at the base of the where it can still grow and function normally. A lingual thyroid can sometimes be mistaken for an overgrown tonsil or tumor in a child and be removed accidentally.

Lymphadenectomy: Term used to describe surgical removal of one or more groups of lymph nodes. It is almost always performed as part of the surgery for cancer. This is usually done because many types of cancer have a tendency to have cancerous cells travel to nearby lymph nodes early in the disease process, this is especially true for thyroid cancer.

Lymphangiogenesis: Is the formation of new lymphatic vessels from pre-existing lymphatic vessels. The process is somewhat similar to angiogenesis but involves lymphatic channels and not blood vessels.

Lymphocytic thyroiditis: Inflammatory disease of the thyroid triggered by a drug or a condition such as pregnancy. Common medications implicated in this process include amiodarone and lithium.

Lymphoma: A type of cancer that begins in the lymphatic cells of the immune system and presents as a solid tumor of lymphoid cells. It is treatable with chemotherapy, and in some cases radiotherapy and/or bone marrow transplantation, and can be curable, depending on the histology, type, and stage of the disease. Thyroid lymphoma is a rare kind of thyroid cancer which can be rapidly growing. Thyroid lymphoma is usually treated not with surgery but with chemotherapy and radiation similar to lymphomas elsewhere in the body.

Magnetic Resonance Imaging (MRI): A common but relatively new radiologic imaging modality used to visualize detailed internal structure and limited function of the body. MRI provides much greater contrast and details between the different soft tissues of the body than computed axial tomography (CAT) does for some body parts especially the brain. MRI uses no ionizing radiation but uses a powerful magnetic field to align hydrogen atoms in water in the body. Radiofrequency fields are used to systematically alter the alignment of this magnetization, causing the hydrogen nuclei to produce a rotating magnetic field detectable by the scanner. This signal can be manipulated by additional magnetic fields to build up enough information to construct an image of the body.

Malignant: Condition synonymous with cancer. Tumors that can progressively worsen with unchecked growth, and develop properties of invasiveness and metastasis and have the potential to result in death. A *malignant tumor* may be contrasted with a noncancerous or benign tumor in that a *malignancy* is not self-limited in its growth, is capable of invading into adjacent tissues, and may be capable of spreading to distant tissues (metastasizing) while a *benign tumor* has none of those properties.

Medullary thyroid cancer: A rare form of thyroid cancer that arises from the parafollicular C-cells of the thyroid gland. C cells are neural-crest derivatives and produce calcitonin. Approximately 25 percent of all medullary thyroid cancers are familial, meaning they occur because of a genetic defect or mutation within a family's lineage that makes that person susceptible to medullary thyroid cancer. The remaining 75 percent occur sporadically, meaning that no one else in the person's family has medullary thyroid cancer and these sporadic cases are usually limited to one side of the thyroid. Patients with certain forms of familial medullary thyroid cancer may need their thyroids removed at a very early age during childhood.

Metabolism: The series of processes by which food is converted into the energy and products needed to sustain life. Metabolism affects body temperature, weight, energy level, muscle strength, mental health, growth, and fertility.

Metastasis: The spread of cancerous cells from one organ or body part to another nonadjacent organ or part. Cancer cells can develop metastatic properties which allow them to break away, leak, or spill from a the main tumor into blood or lymphatic vessels and circulate through the bloodstream. These metastatic circulating tumor cells can then be deposited within normal organs such as bone, lung, or liver elsewhere in the body.

Morbidity rates: A measure of disability or poor health due to any cause such as surgery. Postoperative morbidity may be caused by an unexpected event such as infection, heart attack, stroke, or problems with anesthesia.

Mortality rates: A measure of the number of deaths (in general, or due to a specific cause) in some population, scaled to the size of that population, per unit time. Mortality rate is typically expressed in units of deaths per 1,000 individuals per year; thus, a mortality rate of 9.5 in a population of 100,000 would mean 950 deaths per year in that entire population. Mortality rates from thyroid surgery are very low.

Multicentric: In multiple locations.

Multinodular goiter: A kind of goiter or enlargement of the thyroid gland which contains multiple nodules or lumps. Enlargement of some or all of these nodules can results in compression of adjacent local structures resulting in difficulty in breathing or swallowing.

Mutation: Changes in the DNA sequence in the genes of a cell. Mutations can be caused by radiation, viruses, chemicals, or mistakes during DNA replication. Some mutations are silent and don't cause major changes to the cell but others can be damaging to the cell. Some mutation lead to aberrant growth and can result in cancer.

Myxedema coma: A state of decompensated hypothyroidism. The patient may have lab values identical to a "normal" hypothyroid state, but a stressful event such as severe infection, heart attack, or certain medication precipitates sudden worsening into a state of coma with altered mental status, hypothermia, low blood glucose, low blood pressure, and slowed breathing.

Oncogene: A gene that, when mutated or expressed at high levels, helps turn a normal cell into a tumor cell. Most oncogenes require an additional step, such as mutations in another gene, or environmental factors, such as viral infection, to cause cancer.

Orthotopic: In the anatomically correct position.

Otolaryngologist: Surgeon who specializes in the diagnosis and treatment of diseases of the ear, nose, and throat and head and neck disorders. These doctors undergo surgical training composed of one year in general surgery and four years in otolaryngology—head and neck surgery. Some otolaryngologists perform thyroid surgery.

Ovulation: The process in a female's menstrual cycle (period) by which a mature ovarian follicle ruptures and discharges an ovum (also known as an oocyte, female gamete, or casually as an egg).

Papillary thyroid carcinoma: Papillary thyroid cancer is the most common kind of thyroid cancers (80% of all thyroid neoplasms). The development of papillary thyroid cancer is associated with radiation exposure and autoimmune thyroiditis (Hashimoto's thyroiditis), and typically spreads through the lymphatic networks of the body as opposed to the bloodstream or direct invasion. Papillary thyroid cancers are slow-growing so they are typically diagnosed before spreading to other organs in the body (metastasis). Less than five to ten percent of people with papillary thyroid cancers develop distant metastases with the most common sites being either the lungs or bones.

Parathyroid gland: The parathyroid glands are four or more small glands located on the posterior surface (back side) of the thyroid gland. The parathyroid glands are named for their proximity to the thyroid but serve a completely different role than the thyroid gland. They help precisely regulate the level of calcium in the blood and bones by secreting a special hormone called parathyroid hormone.

Pathologist: Pathologists are doctors who diagnose and characterize disease in living patients by examining biopsies, blood samples, or other bodily fluids. In addition, pathologists interpret medical laboratory tests to help prevent illness or monitor a chronic condition. The vast majority of cancer diagnoses are made by pathologists. Pathologists examine tissue biopsies and fine needle aspiration samples from the thyroid under a microscope to determine if they are benign or cancerous. Some pathologists specialize in genetic testing that can, for example, determine the most appropriate treatment for particular types of cancer. Pathologists also review results of tests ordered or performed by specialists, such as blood tests ordered by an endocrinologist.

Pemberton's Sign: A clinical sign noticed by physicians when a patient with massive enlargement of the thyroid results in compression of the jugular veins draining the head and neck. The sign includes development of facial redness and flushing accompanied by distended superficial neck veins and sometimes resulting in shortness of breath when the patient is asked to raise both arms above his or her head simultaneously, as high as possible (Pemberton's maneuver). This sign is named after Dr. Hugh Pemberton.

Pheochromocytoma: A tumor that originates in the neuroendocrine cells of the adrenal gland but can sometimes grow out of similar cells sitting outside of the adrenal. This kind of tumor is usually non cancerous but can be life threatening as it can secrete excessive amounts of adrenaline (epinephrine) or noradrenaline (norepinephrine). These tumors can be found in some patients with medullary thyroid cancer. Most such patients have a syndrome called multiple endocrine neoplasia syndrome, type IIA (also known as MEN IIA) and type IIB MEN IIB. The other component neoplasms of that syndrome include parathyroid adenomas and medullary thyroid cancer. Mutations in the autosomal RET proto-oncogene drives these malignancies. It is now postulated that U.S. President Abraham Lincoln suffered from MEN IIB, rather than Marfan's syndrome as previously thought, though this is uncertain.

Pituitary gland: A small pea-sized gland in the brain in a small bony pocket called the sella turcica. Located at the base of the brain, the pituitary is composed of two lobes: the anterior pituitary (adenohypophysis) and the posterior pituitary (neurohypophysis). The pituitary is functionally linked to the hypothalamus by the pituitary stalk whereby hypothalamic releasing factors are released and, in turn, stimulate the release of pituitary hormones. Although the pituitary gland is known as the master endocrine gland, both of its lobes are under the control of the hypothalamus. The pituitary gland secretes thyroid stimulating hormone (TSH). If there are problems with the pituitary gland, it can cause problems with the production of many other hormones in the body including thyroid hormone.

Postpartum: Relating to or occurring in the period immediately after childbirth.

Pretibial myxedema: A skin lesion seen in one to four percent of patients with Graves' disease usually presents itself as a waxy, discolored induration, and pitting edema of skin on the shins and top of the foot.

Prevalence: An epidemiologic term which is defined as the total number of cases of the disease in the population at a given time, or the total number of cases in the population, divided by the number of individuals in the population. It is used as an estimate of how common a condition is within a population over a certain period of time. It helps doctors or other health professionals understand the probability of certain diseases such as cancer, including thyroid cancer.

Proto-oncogene: A normal gene that can become an oncogene due to mutations or increased expression. The resultant protein is then called an oncoprotein. Proto-oncogenes code for proteins that help regulate cell growth and differentiation such as molecules involved in cell division or signal transduction. An example of proto-oncogenes important to thyroid cancer is Ras.

Radiologist: Medical doctors that utilize an array of imaging technologies (such as ultrasound, computed tomography (CT), nuclear medicine, positron emission tomography (PET), and magnetic resonance imaging (MRI) to diagnose or treat disease. Interventional radiologist can perform thyroid biopsies or other minimally invasive medical procedures with the guidance of imaging technologies such as an ultrasound.

Radionuclide scanning: A form of nuclear medicine imaging in which radiopharmaceuticals are taken internally, for example intravenously or orally. Then, external detectors (gamma cameras) capture and form images from the radiation emitted by the radiopharmaceuticals. This process is unlike a diagnostic X-ray where external radiation is passed through the body to form an image. These tests generally look at the function of the thyroid gland by measuring how much iodine it can take up from the bloodstream in a set period of time. ^{123}I, a safe but radioactive tagged isotope of iodine, is injected into the bloodstream and accumulates in the thyroid. If one area of the thyroid is producing too much thyroid hormone, this area will show up as a "hot" spot or hot nodule in the pictures of the thyroid taken with a special gamma counter camera. ^{123}I scanning is only used to tell the function of the thyroid after blood tests have shown a suppressed TSH level thus indicating a nodule that may be producing too much thyroid hormone and thus suppressing the TSH level.

Recurrent Laryngeal Nerves: These important paired nerves each branch from the Vagus or Xth cranial nerve. Each nerve supplies sensation to the back of the throat and also helps move the vocal cord muscles on that side. It is referred to as "recurrent" because the branches of the nerve innervate the travel to their final position in the larynx through a rather circuitous route; first it descends into the thoracic cavity before rising up between the trachea and esophagus to reach the neck. Damage to one recurrent laryngeal nerve can result in immobility of one vocal cord and hoarseness. Damage to both recurrent laryngeal nerves can result in difficulty with breathing.

RET proto-oncogene: A proto-oncogene which codes for an important receptor tyrosine kinase. Mutations in this proto-oncogene can result in—medullary thyroid carcinoma, multiple endocrine neoplasias type 2A and 2B, pheochromocytoma, and parathyroid hyperplasia.

Salivary glands: Special exocrine glands that secrete saliva into ducts that empty into the mouth. Salivary glands can be damaged by radioactive iodine because they contain iodine receptors. Damage to these glands can result in a dry mouth and possibly to increased risk of cavities.

Scalpel: A small but extremely sharp bladed instrument used for surgery.

Secondary hyperthyroidism: A form of hyperthyroidism which is very rare and is not due to primary dysfunction of the thyroid itself but caused by either a pituitary tumor or from pituitary resistance to thyroid hormone.

Sodium-iodine symporter (NIS): A special mineral pump present on the surface of thyroid cells that actively transports iodide molecules (I-) across the cell membrane into the thyroid cells. The pump simultaneously moves two sodium ions for every iodide ion. This symporter is driven by a low internal sodium concentration inside the thyroid cells, via facilitated diffusion, caused by another pump called the sodium/potassium ATPase pump. Radiodine treatment used for killing thyroid cancer cells fools the thyroid cells into pumping a radioactive form of iodine into the cell through this surface pump.

Struma ovarii: A rare kind of tumor called a teratoma which contains mostly thyroid tissue. The tumor is made out of embryonic germ cells and most often but not always found in the ovary, these tumors are usually benign and can result in thyrotoxicosis.

Subacute granulomatous thyroiditis: Inflammatory disease of the thyroid, probably caused by infection of the thyroid gland with viral particles. People with this form of sub-acute thyroiditis may present with high fever, malaise joint pains, fatigue, and severe neck pain that may limit their ability to swallow. Thyroid hormone levels are often extremely elevated, resulting in marked signs and symptoms of thyrotoxicosis. This disease is also known as *de Quervain's* thyroiditis.

Subacute thyroiditis: Self-limiting inflammatory thyroid condition that will improve with supportive care only. This form of inflammation is often caused by the body's own immune system attacking the thyroid resulting in release of too much thyroid hormone. Can sometimes be due to an infection in the thyroid and other times due to a particular medication the person might be taking.

Substernal goiter: Enlargement of the thyroid gland which grows below the sternum or breastbone.

Survival rate: Use of biostatistics to figure out the percentage of people in a study or treatment group who are alive for a given period of time after diagnosis. Survival rates are important for prognosis, for example, whether a type of cancer has a good or bad prognosis can be determined from its survival rate. Doctors often use mean overall survival rates to estimate the patient's prognosis. This is often expressed over standard time periods, like one, five, and ten years. For example thyroid cancer has a much better prognosis than pancreatic cancer because five year survival from thyroid cancer is basically close to 95 percent whereas five year survival for pancreatic cancer is closer to five to ten percent. When someone is more interested in how survival is affected by the disease, there is also the net survival rate, which filters out the effect of mortality from other causes than the disease. The two main ways to calculate overall survival are relative survival and disease specific survival. Relative survival is calculated by dividing the overall survival after diagnosis of a disease by the survival as observed in a similar population that was not diagnosed with that disease. A similar population is composed of individuals with at least age and gender similar to those diagnosed with the disease. Disease specific survival is calculated by treating deaths from other causes than the disease as withdrawals from the population that don't lower survival, comparable to patients who are not observed any longer, e.g., due to reaching the end of the study period. Relative survival has the advantage that it does not depend on accuracy of the reported cause of death; disease specific survival has the advantage that it does not depend on the ability to find a similar population of people without the disease.

Symptom: An indication of an illness, disease, or other disorder, especially one experienced by the patient, e.g., pain, dizziness, or itching, as opposed to one observed by the doctor that is considered a sign of the disease or illness.

Targeted therapy: A type of drug developed with the aim of blocking the growth of cancer cells by interfering with specific targeted molecules needed for tumor growth, rather than by simply interfering with rapidly dividing cells (e.g., with traditional chemo-therapy). In theory, targeted cancer therapies may be more effective than current treatments and less harmful to normal cells. Most targeted therapies are either antibodies or small molecules. Many targeted therapies are being developed for tyrosine kinase receptors that are affected in thyroid cancer cells.

Tetany: A medical sign in which involuntary contraction of muscles, caused by diseases and other conditions that increase the action potential frequency. The usual cause of tetany is lack of calcium, this can happen after thyroid surgery if the parathyroids are temporarily stunned or permanently do not work due to altered blood supply.

Thionamide: A class of pharmacologic drugs that are used to control thyrotoxicosis. Two popular thionamides in the United States are methimazole and propylthiouracil.

Thyrogen: A drug, recombinant human TSH (rhTSH) manufactured by a pharmaceutical company called Genzyme. The rhTSH is a synthetic version of thyroid-stimulating hormone (also known as TSH or thyrotropin) and is used in the treatment of some patients with thyroid cancer.

Thyroglobulin: This 660 kDa, dimeric protein is produced and used by the thyroid gland to produce its most important product—thyroid hormone (T3 and T4). Thyroglobulin is produced by the thyroid epithelial cells, which form spherical follicles. Thyroglobulin is secreted and stored in the follicular lumen. Thyroglobyulin is covalently bonded to tyrosine to form monoiodotyrosine (MIT) and diiodotyrosine (DIT). If a person has too much thyroglobulin it usually means there is either inflammation or leakage from the thyroid, the thyroid is very enlarged, or in some cases there is a thyroid cancer which is producing too much thyroglobulin.

Thyroglossal ducts cyst: Usually a cyst in the midline of the upper part of the neck caused by developmental defect in the fetus along the track the thyroid takes during its descent from its original location at the base of the tongue. In the fetus, at three to four weeks of gestation, the thyroid gland appears as an epithelial proliferation in the floor of the pharynx at the base of the tongue in an area called the foramen cecum. The thyroid then descends as a bilobed diverticulum through the thyroglossal duct. Over the next few weeks, it migrates to the base of the neck. During migration, the thyroid remains connected to the tongue by a narrow canal—the thyroglossal duct. Thyroglossal ducts cysts are remnants of this duct and can often present during childhood or early adulthood as an infected lump in the neck but is connected at its most superior aspect to the hyoid bone.

Thyroid follicle: A small anatomical gathering of thyroid epithelia cells with a small cavity in the center where thyroid hormone is stored and later secreted from. The thyroid gland is composed of spherical follicles that selectively absorb iodine (as iodide ions, I⁻) from the blood for production of thyroid hormones. The follicles are surrounded by a single layer of thyroid epithelial cells, which secrete thyroid hormone (T3 and T4). Inside the follicles, the colloid serves as a reservoir of materials for thyroid hormone production and, to a lesser extent, act as a reservoir for the hormones themselves. Scattered among follicular cells and in the spaces between the spherical follicles is another type of thyroid cell, parafollicular cells (also known as C-cells), which secrete another hormone called calcitonin.

Thyroid function tests (TFT): Collection of blood tests used to evaluate function of the thyroid. TFTs may be requested if a patient is thought to suffer from hyperthyroidism (overactive thyroid) or hypothyroidism (underactive thyroid), or to monitor the effectiveness of either thyroid-suppression or hormone replacement therapy.

Thyroid lobectomy (partial thyroidectomy): Surgical removal of one half of the thyroid gland. This is the most minimal thyroid operation in which one half of the thyroid is removed. Patients who have half their thyroid removed usually do not need to take any thyroid hormone post-surgery. This operation is often done if the diagnosis is not clearly a cancer after the fine needle aspiration.

Thyroid nodule: An abnormal growth or lump of thyroid tissue. When they are large or when they occur in very thin individuals, they can even sometimes be seen as a lump in the front of the neck. Thyroid nodules are very common and can range in size from several millimeters to several centimeters. Very large nodules may replace nearly half the thyroid and are visible to the naked eye. Most nodules are noncancerous but some can be malignant. An ultrasound guided fine needle aspiration is currently the most cost-effective, sensitive and accurate way of telling which thyroid nodules harbor cancerous cells.

Thyroid peroxidase (TPO): is an enzyme important for the production of thyroid hormone. This enzyme which is mainly produced in the thyroid gland liberates iodine and allows the iodine to be coupled to tyrosine residues on thyroglobulin for proper production of thyroid hormone.

Thyroid Stimulating Hormone (TSH): A special regulatory hormone secreted by the pituitary gland in the brain which stimulates thyroid hormone production and secretion in the thyroid gland. The level of thyroid hormones (T_3 and T_4) in the blood has an effect on the pituitary release of TSH; when the levels of T_3 and T_4 are low, the production of TSH is increased, and, on the converse, when levels of T_3 and T_4 are high, TSH production is decreased. This effect creates a regulatory negative feedback loop.

Thyroiditis: Inflammation in the thyroid gland. Thyroiditis is generally caused by an attack on the thyroid gland, resulting in inflammation and damage to the thyroid cells. This disease is often considered a malfunction of the immune system with antibodies that attack the cells. It can also be caused by an infection, like a virus or bacteria, which works in the same way as antibodies to cause inflammation in the glands. Some drugs can also cause thyroiditis because they have a tendency to damage thyroid cells.

Thyrotoxicosis factitia: Hyperthyroidism that is induced intentionally or accidentally by short or long-term ingestion of thyroid hormone.

Thyrotoxicosis: Medical condition in which there is clinical effects of excessive thyroid hormone, whether or not the problem is with the thyroid gland itself.

Total thyroidectomy (complete thyroidectomy): Surgical removal of the entire thyroid gland. A total thyroidectomy may be considered when thyroid cancer is highly suspected or there are additional risk factors such as radiation exposure. Some cases of benign thyroid disease, such as thyroiditis, large goiter, multiple thyroid nodules, or Graves' disease, are also treated with total thyroidectomy. When patients are contemplating this procedure they should consider the post-surgery need for lifelong thyroid hormone replacement. While five percent of patients having a partial thyroidectomy may need to take thyroid hormone replacement, all patients having a total thyroidectomy take thyroid hormone pills for the rest of their life.

Toxic nodular goiter (or Plummer's syndrome): A condition that can occur when a hyper-functioning nodule or nodules develop within a longstanding goiter. The hyper-functioning nodule then results in hyperthyroidism. The excess production of thyroid hormone is typically gradual and it may take many years for symptoms to develop. Nuclear medicine imaging of a thyroid gland with toxic nodular disease demonstrates areas of increased uptake, which corresponds to the areas of the gland that are hyperfunctioning.

Trachea: The tube in air-breathing vertebrates that conducts air from the throat to the bronchi, strengthened by incomplete rings of cartilage; otherwise known as the windpipe.

Transgenic animal: An animal whose genetic material has been altered using genetic engineering techniques. New DNA originating from a different species is transferred into an animal, usually at the embryonic stage, giving it modified or novel genes. Transgenic mice are considered genetically engineered organism.

Tyrosine Kinase Receptor: Special receptors present on the surface of normal cells which respond to surrounding growth factors, cytokines, and hormones. Some tyrosine kinases when over activated appear to have a critical role in the development and progression of many types of cancer. Some drug companies have developed special drugs to slow down the signals from these important receptors in certain cancers.

Ultrasonography: A radiologic imaging modality in which high-frequency sound waves are generated and used to view internal organs. The thyroid is a superficial organ in the neck and can be seen very well with ultrasound. Ultrasound is safe and non invasive, does not use any radiation, and is commonly used to detect nodules, cysts, and tumors of the thyroid. Ultrasound is almost always the first imaging test used in patients with thyroid problems because it is very good at looking at growths inside the thyroid gland.

Vagus: This important nerve is the tenth of twelve paired cranial nerves. This nerves exits the brain through the jugular foramen then passing into the carotid sheath between the internal carotid artery and the internal jugular vein where it eventually travels to the thoracic and abdominal cavities. The vagus nerve gives off the recurrent laryngeal nerve on each side.

Wolff-Chaikoff effect: An auto-regulation phenomena in humans who are exposed to high levels of iodine shutting down thyroid hormone production. This was first discovered in 1948 by Drs. Jan Wolff and Israel Lyon Chaikoff at the University of California who noted that increasing blood iodine levels above a certain level caused a shutdown of thyroid hormone production in rats.

Further Reading

THYROID NODULES

American Association of Clinical Endocrinologists: www.aace.com/newsroom/disorders/index.php.

American Thyroid Association: www.thyroid.org/patients/index.html.

Cooper, D. S., Doherty, G. M., Haugen, B. R., Kloos, R. T., Lee, S. L., Mandel, S. J., Mazzaferri, E. L., McIver, B., Sherman, S. I., Tuttle, R. M. Management guidelines for patients with thyroid nodules and differentiated thyroid cancer. American Thyroid Association Guidelines Taskforce. *Thyroid* 2006 Feb;16(2):109–142.

Gharib, H., Papini, E., Valcavi, R., Baskin, H. J., Crescenzi, A., Dottorini, M. E., Duick, D. S., Guglielmi, R., Hamilton, C. R. Jr., Zeiger, M. A., Zini, M. American Association of Clinical Endocrinologists and Associazione Medici Endocrinology medical guidelines for clinical practice for the diagnosis and management of thyroid nodules. AACE/AME Task Force on Thyroid Nodules. *Endocr. Pract.* 2006 Jan–Feb;12(1):63–102.

Hegedüs, L. Clinical practice. The thyroid nodule. *N. Engl. J. Med.* 2004 Oct 21; 351(17):1764–1771.

Izquierdo, R., Arekat, M. R., Knudson, P. E., Kartun, K. F., Khurana, K., Kort, K., Numann, P. J. Comparison of palpation-guided versus ultrasound-guided fine-needle aspiration biopsies of thyroid nodules in an outpatient endocrinology practice. *Endocr. Pract.* 2006 Nov–Dec;12(6):609–614.

McCoy, K. L., Jabbour, N., Ogilvie, J. B., Ohori, N. P., Carty, S. E., Yim, J. H. The incidence of cancer and rate of false-negative cytology in thyroid nodules greater than or equal to 4 cm. in size. *Surgery* 2007 Dec;142(6):837–844.

Tan, G. H., Gharib, H. Thyroid incidentalomas: management approaches to nonpalpable nodules discovered incidentally on thyroid imaging. *Ann. Intern. Med.* 1997 Feb 1; 126(3):226–231.

Yeung, M. J., Serpell, J. W. Management of the solitary thyroid nodule. *Oncologist* 2008; 13(2):105–112.

THYROID FINE NEEDLE ASPIRATION AND THYROID PATHOLOGY

Anton, R. C. Wheeler, T. M. Frozen section of thyroid and parathyroid specimens. *Arch. Pathol. Lab. Med.* 2005;129:1575–1584.

Baloch, Z. W., et al. Diagnostic terminology and morphologic criteria for cytologic diagnosis of thyroid lesions: a synopsis of the National Cancer Institute Thyroid Fine-Needle Aspiration State of the Science Conference. *Diagn. Cytopathol.* 2008;36:425–437.

Castro, M. R., Gharib, H. Thyroid fine-needle aspiration biopsy: progress, practice, and pitfalls. *Endocr. Pract.* 2003;9(2):128–136

LiVolsi, V. A., Baloch, Z. W. Use and abuse of frozen section in the diagnosis of follicular thyroid lesions. *Endocr. Pathol.* 2005;16:285–293.

Pinchot, S. N., Al-Wagih, H., Schaefer, S., Sippel, R., Chen, H. Accuracy of fine-needle aspiration biopsy for predicting neoplasm or carcinoma in thyroid nodules 4 cm or larger. *Arch. Surg.* 2009 Jul;144(7):649–655.

THYROID CARCINOMA

Cooper, D. S., et al. Management guidelines for patients with thyroid nodules and differentiated thyroid cancer. *Thyroid* 2006;16:109–142.

Derringer, G. A., Thompson, L. D., Frommelt, R. A., Bijwaard, K. E., Heffess, C. S., Abbondanzo, S. L. Malignant lymphoma of the thyroid gland: a clinicopathologic study of 108 cases. *Am. J. Surg. Pathol.* 2000 May;24(5):623–639.

Doria, R., Jekel, J. F., Cooper, D. L. Thyroid lymphoma. The case for combined modality therapy. *Cancer* 1994 Jan 1;73(1):200–206.

Fialkowski, E. A., Moley J. F. Current approaches to medullary thyroid carcinoma, sporadic and familial. *J. Surg. Oncol.* 2006;94:737–747.

Graff-Baker, A., Sosa, J. A., Roman, S. Primary thyroid lymphoma: a review of recent developments in diagnosis and histology-driven treatment. *Curr. Opin. Oncol.* epub October 2009.

Green, L. D., Mack, L., Pasieka, J. L. Anaplastic thyroid cancer and primary thyroid lymphoma: a review of these rare thyroid malignancies. *J. Surg. Oncol.* 2006 Dec 15; 94(8):725–736.

Jiménez, C., Hu, MI-N., Gagel, R. F. Management of medullary thyroid carcinoma. *Endocrinol. Metab. Clin. N. Am.* 2008;37:481–496.

Kloos, R. T., Eng, C., Evans, D. B., et al. Medullary thyroid cancer: management guidelines of the american thyroid association. *Thyroid* 2009;19(6):565–612.

Mack, L. A., Pasieka, J. L. An evidence-based approach to the treatment of thyroid lymphoma. *World J. Surg.* 2007 May;31(5):978–986.

Pasieka, J. L. Hashimoto's disease and thyroid lymphoma: role of the surgeon. *World J. Surg.* 2000 Aug;24(8):966–970.

Roman, S., Lin, R., Sosa, J. A. Prognosis of medullary thyroid carcinoma: demographic, clinical, and pathologic predictors of survival in 1252 cases. *Cancer* 2006; 107:2134–2142.

Roman, S., Pritesh, M., Sosa, J. A. Medullary thyroid cancer: early detection and novel treatments. *Curr. Opin. Oncol.* 2008;21:5–10.

THYROID SURGERY

Adler, J. T., Sippel, R. S., Schaefer, S, Chen, H. Preserving function and quality of life after thyroid and parathyroid surgery. *Lancet. Oncol.* 2008;9(11):1069–1075.

Chisholm, E. J., Kulinskaya, E., Tolley, N. S. Systematic review and meta-analysis of the adverse effects of thyroidectomy combined with central neck dissection as compared with thyroidectomy alone. *Laryngoscope* 2009;19(6);1135–1139.

Dralle, H., Machens, A. Surgical approaches in thyroid cancer and lymph-node metastases. *Best Pract. Res. Clin. Endocrinol Metab.* 2008;22(6);971–987.

Garsi, J., et al. Therapeutic Administration of 131I for Differentiated Thyroid Cancer: Radiation Dose to Ovaries and Outcome of Pregnancies. *J. Nucl. Med.* 2008; 49(5):845–852.

Kloos, R. T., et al. Medullary thyroid cancer: Management guidelines of the American Thyroid Association. *Thyroid* 2009;19:565–612.

Mitchell, J., Milas, M., Barbosa, G., Sutton, J., Berber, E., Siperstein, A: Avoidable reoperations for thyroid and parathyroid surgery. Effect of hospital volume. *Surgery* 2008; 144:899–907.

National Comprehensive Cancer Network. NCCN Practice Guidelines in Oncology: Thyroid Carcinoma (v.1.2009): http://www.nccn.org/professionals/physician_gls/f _guidelines.asp.Cooper, D. S., et al. Management Guidelines for Patients with Thyroid Nodules and Differentiated Thyroid Cancer. *Thyroid* 2009, in press.

Pacini F., et al. Radioactive Ablation of Thyroid Remnants after Preparation with Recombinant Human Thyrotropin in Differentiated Thyroid Carcinoma: Results of an Internation, Randomized, Controlled Study. *JCEM* 2006;29(2);926–932.

Remi, H., et al. [131]I Effective Half-Life and Dosimetry in Thyroid Cancer Patients. *J. Nucl. Med.* 2008;49(9):1445–1450.

Saunders, B. D., Wainess, R. M., Dimick, J. B., Doherty, G. M., Upchurch, G. R., Gauger, P.G: Who performs endocrine operations in the United States? *Surgery* 2003; 134:924–931.

Snyder, S. K., et al. Local anesthesia with monitored anesthesia care vs. general anesthesia in thyroidectomy. *Arch. Surg.* 2006;1414:167–173.

Sosa, J. A., Bowman, H. M., Tielsch, J. M., Powe, N. R., Gordon, T. A., Udelsman, R: The importance of surgeon experience for clinical and economic outcomes from thyroidectomy. *Ann. Surg.* 1998;228:320–330.

Spanknebel, K., et al. Thyroidectomy using local anesthesia: A report of 1,025 cases over 16 years. *J. Am. Coll. Surg.* 2005;201:375–385.

Spanknebel, K., et al. Thyroidectomy using monitored local or conventional general anesthesia: An analysis of outpatient surgery, outcome and cost in 1,194 consecutive cases. *World J. Surg.* 2006;30:813–824.

RADIOACTIVE IODINE

Cooper, D. S., et al. Management guidelines for patients with thyroid nodules and differentiated thyroid cancer. *Thyroid* 2009, in press.

Garsi, J., et al. Therapeutic Administration of 131I for Differentiated Thyroid Cancer: Radiation Dose to Ovaries and Outcome of Pregnancies. *J. Nucl. Med.* 2008; 49(5):845–852.

National Comprehensive Cancer Network. NCCN Practice Guidelines in Oncology: Thyroid Carcinoma (v.1.2009): www.nccn.org/professionals/physician_gls/f _guidelines.asp.

Pacini, F., et al. Radioactive Ablation of Thyroid Remnants after Preparation with Recombinant Human Thyrotropin in Differentiated Thyroid Carcinoma: Results of an Internation, Randomized, Controlled Study. *JCEM* 2006;29(2):926–932.

Remy, H., et al. 131 I Effective Half-Life and Dosimetry in Thyroid Cancer Patients. *J. Nucl. Med.* 2008;49(9):1445–1450.

Index

About the Authors

SAREH PARANGI is surgeon at Harvard University's Massachusetts General Hospital. She dedicates her research and clinical practice to patients with thyroid and parathyroid disorders. She is a strong advocate of patient education and strongly advocates that patients be educated and included in all aspects of their own medical care. She did her undergraduate work at Barnard College and obtained her medical degree at Columbia University in New York. She finished her surgical training at the University of California, San Francisco and went on to do important basic science research on how tumors recruit blood vessels. She has won the American Thyroid Association ThyCA Research Award for basic research in thyroid cancer.

ROY PHITAYAKORN is also a surgeon at the Massachusetts General Hospital in Boston, Mass. He did his undergraduate studies at Allegheny College in Meadville, Penn., where he was bestowed with several leadership awards. He was the recipient of the University of Pittsburgh, School of Medicine's Sheehan/Cheke Memorial Prize for Exemplifying the Patient-Physician Relationship in 2002 and also the recipient of the 2002 Healthcare Foundation of New Jersey Humanism in Medicine Student Award. He also has a master's degree in medical education from the University of Illinois in Chicago where he was awarded with the Best Thesis award in the Department of Medical Education in 2008.